Current Clinical Psychiatry

Series Editor

Jerrold F. Rosenbaum
Massachusetts General Hospital, Chief of Psychiatry, Boston, MA

For further volumes:
http://www.springer.com/series/7634

Nhi-Ha Trinh · Yanni Chun Rho ·
Francis G. Lu · Kathy Marie Sanders
Editors

Handbook of Mental Health and Acculturation in Asian American Families

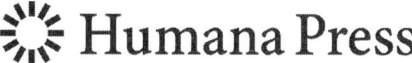

Editors

Nhi-Ha Trinh
Harvard Medical School
Department of Psychiatry
Boston, MA
ntrinh@partners.org

Francis G. Lu
University of California
  at San Francisco
Department of Psychiatry
San Francisco, CA
Francis.Lu@sfdph.org

Yanni Chun Rho
Family, Youth, and Children's Services
Mental Health Division
City of Berkeley
Berkeley, CA, USA
yrho@ci.berkeley.ca.us

Kathy Marie Sanders
Harvard Medical School
Assistant Professor of Psychiatry
Boston, MA
ksanders@partners.org

ISBN 978-1-60327-436-4   e-ISBN 978-1-60327-437-1
DOI 10.1007/978-1-60327-437-1

Library of Congress Control Number: 2008942151

© Humana Press, a part of Springer Science+Business Media, LLC 2009

All rights reserved. This work may not be translated or copied in whole or in part without the written permission of the publisher (Humana Press, c/o Springer Science+Business Media, LLC, 233 Spring Street, New York, NY 10013, USA), except for brief excerpts in connection with reviews or scholarly analysis. Use in connection with any form of information storage and retrieval, electronic adaptation, computer software, or by similar or dissimilar methodology now known or hereafter developed is forbidden.

The use in this publication of trade names, trademarks, service marks, and similar terms, even if they are not identified as such, is not to be taken as an expression of opinion as to whether or not they are subject to proprietary rights.

While the advice and information in this book are believed to be true and accurate at the date of going to press, neither the authors nor the editors nor the publisher can accept any legal responsibility for any errors or omissions that may be made. The publisher makes no warranty, express or implied, with respect to the material contained herein.

Printed on acid-free paper

springer.com

Preface

This volume represents a culmination of a project begun in 2004, planning a nationwide symposium sponsored by the Massachusetts General Hospital (MGH)/McLean Hospital Adult Psychiatry Training Program and the American Psychiatric Association (APA)/SAMHSA (Substance Abuse Mental Health Services Administration) Minority Fellowship Program. Interested in the impact of acculturation on Asian American individuals and their families, we brought together a group of national experts to explore this topic. In the first half of the symposium, researchers discussed the development of acculturation scales, reviewed research on the impact of acculturation on mental health, and presented current research regarding acculturation. In the second half of the symposium, clinicians discussed how to incorporate acculturation in clinical practice, including working with families and special populations such as Southeast Asian Americans. What emerged in November 2005 was a day filled with thoughtful, lively exchange and discussion. The momentum generated from the symposium inspired the conception of this book, a synthesis of the work that was presented that day.

We are fortunate to have this opportunity and would like to thank those who made this symposium and book possible. We are grateful for the support of the APA/SAMHSA Minority Fellowship Program, the MGH Department of Psychiatry, MGH/McLean Hospital Adult Psychiatry Training Program, and the MGH Psychiatry Academy. We were fortunate to have MGH Psychiatry Academy document the symposium and archive it as a webcast on their web site: http://www.mghcme.org (search "Asian" to find our webcasts). We would also like to thank all of our authors for their hard work, generous gift of time, and gracious spirit with which they contributed to this project; our book project sponsor, Dr. Jerrold Rosenbaum, the Chair of the MGH Department of Psychiatry; our editor Mr. Richard Lansing and Humana Press; and Ms. Sara Nadelman, our symposium organizer.

Special thanks go to our co editors Drs. Francis Lu and Kathy Sanders who provided oversight and editorial support from conceptualization to finalization of the symposium and book projects. In particular, Dr. Kathy Sanders, the MGH/McLean Adult Psychiatry Residency Training Director, supported the creative use of the APA/SAMHSA Minority Fellowship and instilled a respect and acceptance of diversity throughout our training experiences. We hope that this book, like that day in November 2005, will foster interest in exploring the role acculturation plays in the mental health of Asian Americans.

Boston, MA	Nhi-Ha Trinh
Berkeley, CA	Yanni C. Rho
San Francisco, CA	Francis G. Lu
Boston, MA	Kathy M. Sanders

Contents

Part I Research on Acculturation in Asian American Mental Health

Acculturation: Measurements and Review of Findings 3
Richard M. Suinn

Theories and Research on Acculturation and Enculturation Experiences among Asian American Families 25
Bryan S.K. Kim, Annie J. Ahn, and N. Alexandra Lam

Strengthening Intergenerational/Intercultural Ties in Immigrant Families (SITIF): A Parenting Intervention to Bridge the Chinese American Intergenerational Acculturation Gap 45
Yu-Wen Ying

Acculturation: Recommendations for Future Research 65
Richard M. Suinn

Part II Clinical Insights on Acculturation in Asian American Mental Health

The Impact of Immigration and Acculturation on the Mental Health of Asian Americans: Overview of Epidemiology and Clinical Implications 81
Siyon Rhee

Assessing Asian American Family Acculturation in Clinical Settings: Guidelines and Recommendations for Mental Health Professionals 99
K.M. Chun and P.D. Akutsu

The A-B-C in Clinical Practice with Southeast Asians: Basic Understanding of Migration and Resettlement History 123
Khanh T. Dinh

Clinical Considerations When Working with Asian American Children and Adolescents 143
Yanni Rho and Kathy Rho

Acculturation and Asian American Elderly 167
Nhi-Ha Trinh and Iqbal Ahmed

Clinical Insights from Working with Immigrant Asian Americans and Their Families: Focus on Acculturation Stressors 179
Nalini V. Juthani and A.S. Mishra

Conclusion 199
Nhi-Ha Trinh and Yanni Rho

Index 201

Contributors

Iqbal Ahmed John A. Burns School of Medicine, University of Hawai'i at Manoa, Honolulu, HI, USA, AhmedI@dop.hawaii.edu

Annie J. Ahn Psychological and Counseling Services, University of San Diego, San Diego, CA, USA

Phillip D. Akutsu Department of Psychology, California State University, Sacramento, Sacramento, CA, USA, akutsu@csus.edu

Kevin M. Chun Department of Psychology, University of San Francisco, San Francisco, CA, USA, chunk@usfca.edu

Khanh T. Dinh Department of Psychology, University of Massachusetts Lowell, Lowell, MA, USA, khanh_dinh@uml.edu

Nalini V. Juthani Scarsdale, NY, USA, nalini.juthani@gmail.com

Bryan S. K. Kim Department of Psychology, University of Hawaii at Hilo, Hilo, HI, USA, bryankim@hawaii.edu

N. Alexandra Lam Department of Counseling, Clinical, and School Psychology, University of California at Santa Barbara, Santa Barbara, CA, USA, alam@education.ucsb.edu

Francis G. Lu University of California, San Francisco, San Francisco, CA, USA, Francis.Lu@sfdph.org

Asha S. Mishra Department of Psychiatry, Virginia Commonwealth School of Medicine, Richmond, VA, USA, Tasmishra@vcu.edu

Siyon Rhee School of Social Work, California State University, Los Angeles, Los Angeles, CA, USA, srhee@calstatela.edu

Kathy Rho Educational Consultant, Boston, MA, USA

Yanni C. Rho Family, Youth, and Children's Services and Adult Services, Mental Health Division at the City of Berkeley; and private practice. Berkeley, CA, USA, yrho@ci.berkeley.ca.us

Kathy M. Sanders MGH/McLean Adult Psychiatry Residency Training Program, Massachusetts General Hospital, Boston MA, USA; McLean Hospital, Belmont MA, USA, ksanders@partners.org

Richard M. Suinn Department of Psychology, Colorado State University, Fort Collins, CO, USA, suinn@lamar.colostate.edu

Nhi-Ha Trinh Depression Clinical Research Program, Department of Psychiatry, Massachusetts General Hospital, Boston, MA, USA, ntrinh@partners.org

Yu-Wen Ying School of Social Welfare, University of California, Berkeley, Berkeley, CA, USA, ywying10@berkeley.edu

Introduction

Yanni Rho and Nhi-Ha Trinh

Why are we devoting an entire volume to the topic of acculturation? Mental health clinicians are becoming increasingly more equipped to perform culturally relevant assessments and provide culturally sensitive treatment recommendations. But as we know, the lives of our clients and patients are complex. Cultural assessment and formulation is the very necessary foundation for the creation of a narrative for our patients; building further awareness of how the patient experiences his or her own world may include a discussion about certain aspects of acculturative change, such as ethnic/racial identity, immigration, acculturation stress, and intergenerational conflict.

Acculturation is both a process and an outcome. As a process, acculturation occurs when two or more cultures meet. Information from the new culture is integrated into an existing cultural schema, and decisions are made regarding what information is valuable and consistent with whom someone believes they are as an individual. As the authors will demonstrate, there is still much work to be done to standardize the concept and definition, to determine what the process entails as well as to understand how it shapes the individual's experience. In this book, there will be several compelling reasons presented for the inclusion of these concepts in our work with Asian Americans. Although some commonalities in the "Asian" experience exist, how each individual processes these experiences and makes it their own is unique and far from predictable.

The process of acculturation has a direct influence on Asian American mental health. We shall explore in depth some of the current research in acculturation as well as how to incorporate these concepts in our clinical work. This volume may be used as a reference, and each chapter will provide a brief outline of what is to be discussed. The first section, *Research on Acculturation in Asian American Mental Health*, describes past and current research as well as future directions for research in acculturation, whereas the second section, *Clinical Insights on Acculturation in Asian American Mental Health*, presents clinical concepts, dilemmas, and recommendations. Several seminal studies and clinical themes are revisited throughout, as each chapter builds upon the last. Read straight through, this book will provide the reader with some of the historical context of acculturation research and the importance of acculturation in clinical practice with Asian Americans. Read by chapter, the book will provide the reader with information on specific topics of interest.

We realize that Asian Americans represent a population with tremendous diversity. It is difficult to generalize the "Asian American" experience as Asian Americans encompass over 30 different subgroups and Pacific Islanders add an additional 21 groups to our discussion. Consideration of all the differences seems a daunting task, as each group and its individuals have their own particular historical and cultural background, not to mention tremendous diversity in migration history, socioeconomic status, educational background, and family structure. Nevertheless, what we plan to convey through these chapters is a conceptual framework to help guide researchers and clinicians and provide a deepened understanding of acculturation in Asian Americans. The editors and authors are very aware that to discuss all of the many differences among the different ethnicities that fall under the umbrella of "Asian" would take much more than this book will offer. Still, recognizing common themes that are generally relevant to the Asian experience is valuable. These theories or concepts may be incorporated into all clinical work, be it an initial clinical evaluation, ongoing therapy, consultation, or medication management. Each author will highlight some common issues as well as contribute further thoughts and observations specific to certain populations; in addition, some will include original hypotheses and research. And many will further consider the challenges relevant to psychiatric research and clinical practice for Asian American mental health.

Resiliency and strength-based assessment will be referred to throughout this volume. The ability to stand strong and healthy in the face of obstacles and misfortunes is something that we tend to overlook in our clinical worlds. Not all Asian Americans will struggle with mental health issues; not all falter in the face of adverse conditions. There is value in recognizing the particular strengths present in the Asian American population and its individuals, especially given the stigma and shame that is associated with seeking help. Recognizing and reinforcing strengths, such as commitment to family and the ability to successfully navigate between two disparate cultures, may also help build trust and provide affirmation to those with whom we work. Much still needs to be done with regard to formal research on resiliency in Asian populations, but many of the authors do provide suggestions and cite literature that will help guide clinicians and researchers alike in thinking about how to incorporate more strength-focused work into their work with immigrant populations.

Finally, we want to acknowledge that much of the language we use when discussing ethnicity and race is imperfect and imprecise. We use "European American" throughout this publication to represent the ethnic history of those we typically consider "White" while acknowledging that it may inaccurately describe some who are from non-European descent. In addition, some authors have chosen to use words such as "Native country," "Home country," or "Country of origin" to describe the country and culture with which people feel most familiar and connected or to describe the country from which their families originated. Fallible and evolving vocabulary aside, we hope our readers will look past the terms used and find value in the information presented. Our expectation is that this volume will further the increasingly sophisticated discussion of how to best care for our patients and their families and provide a "next step" to the never-ending journey toward clinical and research excellence.

Part I
Research on Acculturation in Asian American Mental Health

Acculturation: Measurements and Review of Findings

Richard M. Suinn

Abstract Acculturation is a process that occurs when two or more cultures interact together. This opening chapter discusses the evolution of the definition of acculturation and identifies scales used to measure acculturation through behavior, values, or a combination of both. The chapter then provides a detailed review of the research literature on the effect of acculturation on Asian Americans, specifically as it pertains to physical health, mental health, school performance, choice of careers, and attitudes toward counseling and therapy.

Keywords Acculturation · Scales · Asian-American mental health · Asian-American physical health · Asian-American school performance · Asian-American careers · Asian-American therapy attitude

Contents

Definition	4
Assessment	5
Behavioral Acculturation Scales: Scales Based on Determining Acculturation by Behaviors	5
Values Acculturation Scales: Scales Based on Determining Acculturation by Values	6
Behavioral and Values Acculturation Scales: Scales Based on Assessment of Behaviors and Values	7
Pan-Ethnic Acculturation Scales: Scales Suitable for Diverse Ethnic Populations	7
Why Study Acculturation—Research Findings	8
Acculturation Status and Physical Health	9
Acculturation Status and Mental Health	11
Acculturation Status and School Performance	14
Acculturation Status and Career Decisions	15
Acculturation Status and Attitudes Toward Counseling and Therapy	16
Summary	18
References	18

R.M. Suinn (✉)
Department of Psychology, Colorado State University, Fort Collins, CO 80523, USA
e-mail: suinn@lamar.colostate.edu

Definition

"Acculturation" has been defined in various ways. An early definition of acculturation was offered by Redfield et al. [1] as "those phenomena which results when groups of individuals sharing different cultures come into continuous first-hand contact, with subsequent changes in the original culture patterns of either or both groups..." (1, p. 149). Leininger [2] suggested that acculturation is the process by which an individual or group from culture A learns how to take on the values, behaviors, norms, and lifestyle of culture B. Berry [3] writes that acculturation is the "process by which individuals change, both by being influenced by contact with another culture and by being participants in the general acculturative changes under way in their own culture" (p. 235). Suinn [4] provides a more simple definition that acculturation is a process that can occur when two or more cultures interact together.

In all of these definitions, acculturation is viewed as a process of change leading to certain outcomes. Initially, acculturation was conceptualized mainly as a linear, unidimensional process, with the process occurring on a continuum. On this continuum, the original culture and the new culture are seen at opposite ends. Within this linear, unidimensional framework, the acculturation process is said to start with "low acculturation" and move toward "high acculturation." Put in other terms, "high acculturation" refers to adoption of the host culture's attitudes, values, or behaviors, whereas "low acculturation" refers to the retention of the culture of origin's characteristics. This model assumes that increments of involvement in the new culture necessarily involve corresponding decrements of involvement with the culture of origin.

A revised perspective expands the view of what the possible outcomes might entail. Instead of a single, linear continuum, a multilinear model focuses on a person's position on both the original culture's and the new culture's norms. Involvement in one society does not necessitate a decrease in involvement in another; therefore, a more comprehensive picture would describe individuals' positions relative to their original cultures' as well as to the new culture's identifying characteristics [5, 6]. This is best illustrated with a person whose culture of origin is Asian, immigrating to a Western country. One possible outcome of such exposure might be that this person retains the Asian cultural characteristics and adopts none of the Western characteristics—in effect showing high Asian and low Western identity. In Berry's terms, this outcome is called *separation*. Another potential outcome might involve loss of Asian attitudes, behaviors, values, and full adoption of Western characteristics—thus showing low Asian and high Western features. Berry would refer to this as *assimilation*. Still, yet a third outcome might include the retention of Asian besides the adoption of Western qualities—thereby showing high Asian as well as high Western characteristics, in other words, a person who is bicultural or at Berry's stage of *integration*. Finally, another outcome could be a rejection of one's prior culture as well as rejection of the Western culture—showing low Asian and low

Western characteristics; in other words, a person who is alienated from both cultures and is *marginalized* according to Berry.[1]

In this chapter, "acculturation" refers to the *process*; the terms "low acculturation" and "high acculturation" refer to the outcomes of the acculturation process; the former refers to the retention of the culture of origin's values, attitudes, and behaviors and the latter refers to the adoption of the host culture's values, attitudes, and behaviors. In addition, in this chapter, the term "Asian-identified" is equivalent to "low acculturation", whereas "Western-identified" is equivalent to "high acculturation" [4].

Assessment

Moyerman and Forman [7], in their definition of acculturation, identify the areas of change as attitudes, behaviors, or values. Similarly, Lee [8] describes acculturation as a process by which consumers learn values, attitudes, and behaviors different from their culture of origin. Also Berry et al. [6] defined the changes as involving cultural behaviors and values that individuals experience as a result of contact between two cultures. Over the years, measures of acculturation status for Asian or Asian-American populations have typically addressed one or both of the following: (a) assessment of acculturation through measuring behaviors or through measuring values or (b) development of a scale that is appropriate for diverse cultures rather than being specifically worded for one or a few cultures. There has also been attention to designing a scale or scoring systems that enable the assessment of individuals' status or commitment to both their country of origin and the host culture's behaviors, attitudes, or values—these are often referred to as orthogonal scales or orthogonal scoring. The following sections will briefly describe a sample of self-administered acculturation scales applicable to Asian or Asian-American populations. For the scales themselves, please refer to the Appendix.

Behavioral Acculturation Scales: Scales Based on Determining Acculturation by Behaviors

The Suinn–Lew Asian Self-Identity Acculturation Scale (SL-ASIA) is a 21-item instrument in which respondents rate the items on a scale from 1 to 5, with low scores representing high-Asian identification and high scores representing high-Western identification [9, 10]. These original 21 items covered behaviors

---

[1] The term acculturation is sometimes used in writings to refer to the process, but also at times to the outcome of the process. Hence, "acculturation" might be used to refer to the outcome whereby an individual adopts the behaviors and values of the host culture as a result of exposure to that culture. On the other hand, "unacculturated" might be used to refer to an individual who retains the behaviors or values of the country of origin.

involving language, friendship choice, food preferences, media preferences, participation in cultural activity, ethnic identity, and geographical and generational history. Although viewed as a linear, unidimensional scale, an orthogonal scoring system is available [11, 12]. In addition, five new items have been developed that not only measure orthogonal information regarding the level of commitment to Asian as well as to Western norms but also cover the topics of values, perceived behavioral competency/comfort, and core self-identity [4]. Several authors have identified the SL-ASIA scale as the 'most widely used scale for measuring Asian-Americans' acculturation levels' [13–16].

The Marin Acculturation Scale, revised [17] is actually a scale originally developed by Marin et al. [18] for Hispanic populations. Gupta and Yick administered it to a group of foreign-born Chinese-Americans to determine its appropriateness and concluded that it could be a valid method. The scale is made up of 12 items regarding the following behaviors: language spoken at home, preference of the ethnicity of people at social gatherings, and language preferred in media. They reported suitable validity results from factor analysis and correlation with the length of residence in the United States.

Values Acculturation Scales: Scales Based on Determining Acculturation by Values

The Asian Values Scale (AVS) contains 36 statements that measure commitment to various Asian cultural values, including collectivism, conformity to norms, emotional self-control, filial piety, humility, and family recognition through achievement [19]. Respondents use a 7-point Likert scale, ranging from "strongly disagree" to "strongly agree." Scores from the AVS were correlated against scores from the SL-ASIA, with the result of $r = 0.15$. Because the AVS was designed as a measure of values, whereas the SL-ASIA assesses behaviors, this low correlation confirmed that the two scales measure different aspects of acculturation. The original AVS has been shortened to a 25-item version, named the Asian Values Scale-Revised [20]. This has been followed by a 42-item version—the Asian-American Values Scale-Multidimensional—that provides subscale scores on the values of collectivism, conformity, emotional self-control, humility, and family recognition [21].

The European American Values Scale for Asian Americans (EAVS-AA) was developed to independently measure Asian-American individuals' adherence to European American values [22]. The authors recognized that the AVS assesses the level of adherence to Asian values and wanted the EAVS-AA to correspondingly assess adherence to European American values to provide a more comprehensive picture. The initial values items were derived from a survey of 369 items, then reduced to 180 items, and finally reduced to a final pool of 18 items on which European Americans scored significantly higher than Asian Americans. Respondents rate each item on a 7-point scale, ranging from "strongly disagree" to "strongly agree." A psychometrically improved 25-item version using a 4-point rating scale has replaced the initial EAVS-AA and is named the European American Values Scale for Asian Americans-Revised (EAVS-AA-R) [23].

Behavioral and Values Acculturation Scales: Scales Based on Assessment of Behaviors and Values

The Acculturation Scale, originally entitled The Acculturation Scale for Vietnamese Adolescents (ASVA), consists of 76 items representing behaviors and values associated with everyday lifestyle, group interactions, family orientation, and traditions [24]. A 5-point scale is used to indicate the respondents' level of agreement with each item. Behavioral items include items such as language, social group, and media preferences. Values items include values such as collectivism/individualism and culturally defined gender roles. Two subscale scores are derived: the IVN (Involvement in the Vietnamese culture) reflects the level of involvement in the Vietnamese culture and the IUS (Involvement in the American culture) score reflects the level of involvement in the US culture. A brief 50-item version is also available [24].

Pan-Ethnic Acculturation Scales: Scales Suitable for Diverse Ethnic Populations

The Asian American Multidimensional Acculturation Scale (AAMAS) is based on the SL-ASIA, but converted into a format appropriate for diverse ethnic populations [13]. The format revision asks respondents to rate each item according to three reference groups: (a) their culture of origin, (b) other Asian Americans, and (c) European Americans. Three subscales result from this approach: AAMAS Culture of Origin, AAMAS-Asian American, and AAMAS-European American. Each subscale is composed of 15 items assessing cultural behaviors, cultural knowledge, and cultural identity. Responses are rated through a 6-point scale from "not very much" to "very much."

The Stephenson Multigroup Acculturation Scale was designed to be appropriate for persons from diverse ethnic groups and has been tested among groups such as African Americans, Asian Americans (such as Cambodians, East Indians, and Filipinos), European Americans, and Hispanic Americans (such as Brazilians, Mexicans, and Peruvians) [25]. Two subscale scores are derived, representing immersion in the host society and immersion in one's ethnic society. There are a total of 32 items covering language, social interactions, cultural knowledge, food, and media preferences. Respondents use a 4-point scale ranging from "false" to "partly false," "partly true," and "true." The 32 items are in the form of statements, such as "I know how to read and write in my native language" and "I regularly read an American newspaper."

The Acculturation, Habits, and Interests Multicultural Scale for Adolescents (AHIMSA) is available for adolescents from diverse ethnic origins [26]. There are eight items covering food, media, social interactions, and identity. Each item is actually an incomplete statement, such as "I am most comfortable being with people from..." and "The way I do things and the way I think about things are from..." Four answer choices are offered: (a) the United States, (b) the country my family is from, (c) both, and (d) neither. From these answers, four scores are generated based on the four orientations: Assimilation (the total number of "United States" responses), Separation (the total number of "The country my family is from" responses), Integration (the total number of "Both" responses), and Marginalization (the total number of "Neither" responses).

The Multicultural Acculturation Scale (MAS) is made up of items covering behaviors, identity, and values [27]. The MAS includes 24 items involving daily, cultural, and work activities, social interactions, religion and language, and identity. Using a 5-point scale, respondents rate the extent to which their characteristics on these items are like those typical of their culture of origin. A second set of ratings uses the same items but with the referent being the Anglo (Western) culture. Three scores are reported: Ethnic Orientation Index (EOI), Anglo-American Orientation Index (AOI), and an Overall Acculturation Index (OAI). The OAI is calculated by subtracting the EOI from the AOI. A positive score is indicative of assimilation, a negative of separation. A near-zero OAI combined with high EOI and high AOI is interpreted as biculturalism. A near-zero OAI combined with low EOI and low AOI is interpreted as marginality.

The Orthogonal Cultural Identification Scale [16, 28, 29] consists of six basic questions assessing cultural behaviors, self-estimate of success in cultural involvement, and the level of adoption of an identified culture's "way of life." The scale asks participants to rate themselves on each of the six questions consisting of five referent points. For instance, one basic question is "Do you live by or follow the....way of life?" This question is repeated five times, with a different referent group, for example, "Do you live by or follow the White American way of life?" and "Do you live by or follow the Asian American way of life?" The five referent groups are African American, Asian American, American Indian, Mexican American or Spanish, and White American. Ratings are on a 4-point scale from "a lot" to "not at all." Within this model, participants can be assessed regarding their level of acculturation across any pairings of cultures.

Why Study Acculturation—Research Findings

Over the years, an impressive array of research has accumulated, which confirm either the direct or indirect relationship of acculturation outcomes to important variables. Thus, acculturation status has been found associated with physical health, mental health, school performance, and family/marital adjustment. Furthermore, acculturation status has been shown to affect career and personal counseling/psychotherapy processes. The following sections will illustrate such findings from a sample of scholarly studies.

Acculturation Status and Physical Health

Coronary heart disease: Among the classic early findings bringing attention to the role of culture and health are the epidemiologic studies on coronary heart disease (CHD) and stroke among Japanese populations. Prevalence and incidence of CHD were compared among Japanese men residing in Japan, Hawaii, and California. The prevalence rates for definite and possible CHD showed a clear pattern of increasing prevalence from those in Japan to those in Hawaii to those in California, the prevalence rates being 25.4, 34.7, and 44.6, respectively. A similar gradient was also found for the prevalence of angina pectoris and elevated serum cholesterol [30]. Researchers conclude that there is a striking increase in CHD in Japanese who migrate to the United States, with this increase being more pronounced in California than in Hawaii. For instance, the incidence of myocardial infarction and death from CHD among Japanese men in California was nearly 50% greater than that of Japanese men in Hawaii [31].

The Canadian National Population Health survey examined 1,972 Asian immigrants to Canada with respect to the prevalence of hypertension [32]. Findings showed that rates of hypertension increased along with increased years of residence in Canada. This finding was found when other risk factors were controlled, such as smoking, health status and access, drinking, stress, and socioeconomic level. In all these studies, a major conclusion is that exposure to the Western culture—and presumably adoption of the Western lifestyle—is associated with major risk of CHD.

Eating disorders and obesity: Studies have reported on the possible relationship between adopting Western attitudes and values about physical appearance and eating disorders. Mau [33] studied acculturation levels and eating disorder symptoms among 396 Hong Kong schoolgirls. Instruments used were the SL-ASIA, the Eating Attitudes Test (EAT), and the Eating Disorder Inventory (EDI) [34, 35]. Results indicated that girls who were more Westernized scored higher on the EAT and on the bulimia symptoms subscale of the EDI. In a dissertation study, Doan [36] contacted 188 East Asian female undergraduates in the United States to determine the influence of acculturation on eating disorder symptoms. The group of women in the assimilation group showed the highest number of anorexic symptoms as compared with the women in the separation and marginalization groups. In addition, those students who internalized Western attitudes about physical appearances were most symptomatic compared with the rest of the sample. Finally, when all risk factors were controlled, acculturation status continued to contribute to anorexia symptomatology. Using an international sample of students from Hong Kong, Japan,

People's Republic of China, and Taiwan studying in the United States, Stark-Wroblewski et al. [37] also confirmed that the internalization of Western appearance norms was positively associated with eating disorder symptoms.

Unger et al. [38] studied behaviors leading to obesity. They examined the frequency of fast food consumption and of physical fitness activities among Asian American and Hispanic 6th and 7th grade adolescents. Acculturation status was assessed with the AHIMSA. Results showed that acculturation measured in the 6th grade was significantly associated with higher frequency of fast food consumption and a lower frequency of participation in physical fitness activity in the 7th grade. An interesting study by Yang [39] focused on the possible contribution of acculturation distress on emotional eating and hence body weight. Participants were Hmong and Hmong-Americans attending a US college. Results supported the hypothesis that acculturation stress levels were associated with emotional eating behaviors, although acculturation status was not. In addition, a small positive correlation was found between emotional eating and body weight ($r = 0.19$, $P<0.05$), indicating that greater emotional eating was somewhat associated with higher body weight.

Smoking behaviors: In the same way that certain behaviors may be a risk factor for obesity and poor health, smoking is a well-known risk factor for poor physical health. A number of studies have examined the extent to which cultural norms influence smoking behaviors [40, 41]. Of interest are the variable findings of studies on acculturation status and smoking behaviors. One set of research supports the contention that low acculturation among Asians is associated with higher smoking. For instance Ma et al. [42] found low acculturation to be predictive of smoking among a sample of 1,374 Chinese, Cambodians, Koreans, and Vietnamese adult males living in the United States. Similarly, Hofstetter et al. [43] reported that less acculturated adult male Koreans in California reported higher current and predicted future rates of smoking. On a younger sample of 106 Asian-American high-school students, Weiss and Garbanati [44] found that lower acculturation was associated with smoking.

On the other hand, another series of studies report that higher acculturation rather than lower acculturation is associated with higher smoking prevalence rates [45, 46]. Chen et al.'s finding was based on a study of 1,810 Chinese-, Filipino-, Japanese-, and Korean-Americans in California. Unger et al.'s finding came from the Independent Evaluation of the California Tobacco Control, Prevention, and Education Program, which evaluated 15,938 youths. Of these, 4,352 were Hispanic and 3,021 were Asian American. The relevant finding focused on the association between the use of English and smoking behaviors. Results were that speaking only English at home doubled the risk of lifetime smoking compared with students who reported speaking only or mostly another language. As language usage has been accepted as one index of acculturation status, this study would confirm the suggestion that high acculturation is predictive of higher smoking.

There are several possible hypotheses regarding these apparently contradictory findings. One possible explanation is the difference in age groups. The samples of Ma et al. [42] and Hofstetter et al. [43] were adult males, whereas the Chen/Unger series involved youth. Thus, Ma et al. [42] found that less-acculturated male adults but more-acculturated youth had higher smoking rates. Another hypothesis takes into account the context within which the individuals live and how these might interact with the level of acculturation. For instance, Unger and Chen [47] concluded that the surrounding social networks of adolescents have a major influence on smoking. Specifically, the age of initiation of smoking was earlier among adolescents whose friends, siblings, or parents were smokers. Another cross-cultural study by Unger et al. confirmed this finding [48]. Using survey data on 5,780 adolescents in California and 6,992 adolescents in Wuhan, China, the role of friends who smoke was studied. For both cultures, the association with friends who smoke was associated with smoking prevalence, and the strength of this relationship was similar between the two cultures. An additional study conducted by Weiss and Garbanati [44] discovered that what differentiated their Asian-American adolescents who smoked from nonsmokers was lower acculturation plus having a father who smoked.

Alcohol consumption: Alcohol consumption is another risk factor for health. Results have been similar to the prior findings regarding smoking behaviors. Hahm et al. [49] accessed a subsample of the National Longitudinal Adolescent Health data set looking at 714 Asian American adolescents. Asian American adolescents with the highest level of acculturation (English use at home, born in the United States) were identified as the highest risk group. However, a familial factor acted as a further influence. Thus, for adolescents with low parental attachment, the odds of alcohol use were 11 times greater in the higher acculturated group than in the lower acculturated group. Hendershot et al. [50] reported that acculturation and parents' use of alcohol significantly predicted drinking behavior. In addition, Hahm et al. [51] first found that high acculturation level was associated with high binge drinking. However, with further analyses, they concluded that the influence of friends who drink is the important pathway leading to binge drinking. Thus, acculturation status might be considered the first level of variables involved in alcohol consumption, but it is modified by the social or familial context.

Acculturation Status and Mental Health

Psychological distress: Berry has observed that the acculturation process can be stressful to a person struggling to adapt to the new cultural environment. Among the sources of stress facing the new arrival include acquiring a new language to communicate, developing work skills, understanding the new social and behavioral norms, and coping with social isolation and possible racism [52–57]. A number of studies provide concrete information regarding the nature of the relationship between acculturation and stress. Sodowsky and Lai [58] studied 200 immigrants who were Asian Indian, Chinese, Filipino, Japanese,

Korean, or Vietnamese. Acculturation status was significantly related to acculturation stress; the lower the level of acculturation, the higher the distress. Wang and Mallinkrodt [59] surveyed Chinese international students regarding acculturation, anxiety, and psychological symptoms or distress. The specific anxiety measured—"attachment anxiety"—involves worries about being alone and anxiety about being separated from significant figures. Results showed that low Western acculturation was in fact associated with high attachment anxiety. In addition, high levels of attachment anxiety were associated with high psychological symptoms/distress.

Wilton and Constantine [60] examined the cultural distress of 190 Asian and Latin American international college students. They found that the length of residence in the United States was negatively associated with acculturative distress, with higher stress reported by those more recently exposed to the United States. Of interest is the additional finding that students with concerns over their intercultural competency reported higher levels of distress. Lee et al. [61] also examined the relative roles of acculturation, acculturation stress, and mental health symptoms. In 319 Asian immigrant students in junior and senior high schools, acculturation stress was found to be associated with higher mental health symptoms. Furthermore, Asian youths who were more Asian-identified tended to report more mental health symptoms than youths who were more American-identified. Similarly, Ryder et al. [62] found that among Chinese undergraduate students, higher levels of assimilation predicted lower levels of distress, depression, reported symptoms, and social maladjustment.

In addition, several studies are expanding to ask the question of whether acculturation stress can be moderated. For instance, Lee et al. [61] first confirmed that acculturative stress was associated with mental health symptoms among 74 Korean international students in Pennsylvania. However, the availability of social support significantly reduced reports of mental health symptoms even with increased levels of stress. This buffering effect was especially prominent where there was a high level of acculturation skills, such as language. Earlier, Chung et al. [63] compared the levels of psychological distress of immigrant groups arriving in different years. The groups experiencing lower distress were more acculturated and felt they received helpful social support.

Depression and suicide: Although acculturation status has some relationship to depression, this relationship is complex. Shen and Takeuchi [64] examined the role of acculturation on depression with 983 Chinese-American employees, most of whom were immigrants. They discovered that higher levels of acculturation were associated with elevated depressive symptoms, but this was because higher acculturation status involved higher stress levels. However, this relationship between high acculturation and depression was dramatically altered in the presence of other variables. For employees with higher socioeconomic status, better social support, and lower stress, higher acculturation status was associated instead with lower depressive symptoms. Another interesting study is that of Kim et al. [65]. They utilized Berry's proposal that there are four possible outcomes of the acculturation process: assimilation, integration, separation, and marginalization (as defined earlier) [6]. Participants were 60 Chinese-, Japanese-, or Korean-American adolescents, along with 60 mothers and 54 fathers living in California. Most parents immigrated as adults, whereas most adolescents were US born. The results confirmed that parents and adolescents who experience marginalization reported experiencing more intense depressive symptoms. Crane et al. [66] adopted a different point of analysis by examining the interaction between adolescents' acculturation status difference from their parents and depression. Their sample involved 41 adolescents and their parents living in the United States and Canada. They found that when adolescent depression was present, the crucial contributing factor was the existence of discrepancies between the adolescents and their parents in levels of acculturation. Lau et al. [67] conducted a similar analysis to determine whether family variables interacted with acculturation level. They researched suicidal behaviors documented in mental health outpatient clinic records of 285 Asian American youths in California. Less acculturated youths were found to be at greater risk of suicidal behaviors. Under further analysis, an important mediating variable was found to be family conflict. Less-acculturated Asian youths were at greater risk of suicidality under conditions of high parent–child conflict.

Family adjustment: With the high value afforded family matters in the Asian culture, research regarding acculturation and family adjustment assumes importance. Fu [68] contacted 150 Chinese Americans to determine the relationship between acculturation levels and family conflicts. Participants described their acculturation levels and then did the same on behalf of their parents. Results showed that the disparity between acculturation levels was related to family conflict. In a similar approach, Nguyen [69] obtained data from 91 Vietnamese-Americans in California. As with Fu's procedure, participants assessed their own acculturation status on a questionnaire and then completed the same items as they perceived their parents would answer the questions. Results indicated that the greater the difference in acculturation levels between the participants and their ratings of their parents, the higher the likelihood and seriousness of family conflicts. Pyke [70] expanded her study's focus to study siblings' acculturation level differences. Through interviews, she concluded that first-born children tended to be more traditional, whereas younger were more assimilated. These differences, she concluded, tended to be the sources of familial conflict. Sharir [71] also studied the influence of intergenerational discrepancies regarding acculturation with an emphasis on acculturation strategies. For instance, differences were examined where a family member endorsed integration, whereas another endorsed separation. Results confirmed that greater family conflict existed where adolescents adopted a different acculturation strategy compared with their parents. Ying and Han [72] conducted a longitudinal study of 490 Southeast Asian adolescents and confirmed that intergenerational discrepancy predicted intergenerational family conflict 3 years later. In addition, intergenerational conflict was predictive of depressive symptoms.

Acculturation Status and School Performance

There is a perception that Asian students tend to do well academically [73, 74]. In fact, a number of studies lend credence to this perception. In a longitudinal design, Huntsinger et al. [75] compared 40 European American and 40 second-generation Chinese-American preschool and kindergarten children over three testing periods: 1993, 1995, and 1997. The Chinese-American children outscored the European American children in mathematics all three times. Initially, the European American children scored higher than the Chinese children on receptive English vocabulary, but the Chinese children caught up by the third testing and surpassed the European American children in reading by that date. Fuligni et al. [76] conducted their study on high school students of European American, Mexican, or Chinese heritage. They found that commitment to one's ethnic culture was a factor associated with academic achievement. The authors not only concluded that high identification with one's cultural background was associated with high academic achievement among the Mexican and Chinese students, but cultural identification also signified higher academic motivation as well. Such students were more positive about education in general, found school interesting, and believed schooling to be useful for their future.

As with other findings demonstrating the important influence of acculturation status, how acculturation impacts school performance is being discovered. Here, the role of parents seems prominent. Huntsinger et al. [75] concluded that parental involvement, such as requiring more homework, was a significant influence on their children's high mathematics performance. Dandy and Nettelbeck [77] surveyed 239 Australian parents from Chinese, Vietnamese, and European Celtic heritage to identify parental expectations for their children. Results indicated that the Asian parents revealed higher aspirations and higher academic standards for their children's education than the European Celtic parents. Such high expectations were confirmed by a number of researchers using data from the US National Educational Longitudinal Study. The National Longitudinal Study [78] was a survey that included 3,009 African Americans, 1,527 Asian Americans, 16,317 European Americans, 3,171 Mexican Americans, and 299 Native Americans. From this data set, Shin [79] (see also Goyette and Xie, 80; Peng and Wright, 81) concluded that Asian American parents had higher educational expectations for their children than Mexican Americans or European American parents, and that this difference led to the Asian children's superior school performance.

Further research has taken the logical extension of asking how the students themselves viewed academic work, as this might moderate the influence of their parents' high expectations. For instance, if these students believed that success was a function of innate ability, then such a belief would reduce the impact of parental expectations and pressure. What has been found, however, is that Asian American students attribute academic success to factors within their control. For example, Mizokawa and Ryckman [82] asked 4th–11th grade

Asian American students (Chinese, Filipino, Japanese, Korean, and Vietnamese) to what they attribute success or failure in academic work. This sample of over 2,500 students rated effort more than ability as the explanation for academic performance. Similarly, Hau and Salili [83] confirmed that Chinese high school students rated effort, interest in studying, study skill, and the ability in studying to be the most important sources for academic success. Extending the study sample to undergraduate and graduate students, Yan and Faier [84] obtained the responses of 358 European, Chinese, Japanese, Korean, and Southeast Asian American participants. When compared with Asian American students, the European American students attributed academic achievement more to ability than did their Asian American counterparts. On the other hand, Asian American students emphasized effort when identifying the cause for academic achievement or failure. In effect, Asian cultural beliefs and values significantly impact on school performance. Among the important Asian beliefs are the role of hard work and discipline, even at an early age. Also important is the belief that "ability" is accomplished through effort and work, and that achievement precedes ability. In contrast, the European American culture places a greater emphasis on ability in academic achievement and on the belief that ability precedes achievement [85–88]. The research summarized in this section not only documents the influence of Asian parents but also confirms the lasting influence on the beliefs held by the children themselves. A possible conclusion that many Asian families might reach is that when there is academic failure, there is a lack of effort on the child's part, or if more Westernized, a lack of ability. This may be important to consider in a biopsychosocial formulation when working with children and their parents.

Acculturation Status and Career Decisions

Although there are only a small number of studies on acculturation and career decisions, there are some trends in results. Those with high Asian identification appear to select careers that have been stereotyped vocations for Asians (science or numbers oriented). They may place personal interests secondary and follow directions influenced by parental wishes. Tang et al. [89] reported this exact finding on a sample of 187 Asian American college students, concluding that lower acculturation participants chose more Asian-stereotyped occupations and were influenced by their families rather than by their personal interests. Castelino replicated these findings in his study [90]. Whereas Tang et al. involved predominantly Chinese, Vietnamese, and Filipinos born or raised in the United States, Castelino's sample was South Asian participants from Bangladesh, India, Nepal, Pakistan, and Sri Lanka. Once more, the results confirmed that low acculturation participants selected more stereotyped occupations; on the other hand, high acculturation participants expressed interest and choices among more nontraditional, broader sets of occupations. Hsieh [91] studied a slightly different view of the role of acculturation. She looked at the decision-making self-efficacy of 280 Asian American female undergraduates as it might be affected by acculturation level. The level of acculturation was found associated with gender role traditionality; in turn, gender role traditionality directly influenced career decision-making self-efficacy. Finally, low self-efficacy was significantly associated with greater indecision about careers.

As Asian cultural values emphasize commitment to family and respect for parents, it is not surprising that such values influence career decision-making. Tang [92] examined Chinese students in China as well as Asian American and European American college students in the United States. Topics were students' career choices and parental involvement, such as parental career choices for their children and parental involvement in career planning. Results showed that the Chinese and Asian American students were more likely than the European American students to comply with their parental career choices for them. Corey [93] examined the career aspiration of second-generation Asian American college students and concluded that their tendency toward science/numerical career paths was substantially influenced by their perception of their parents' aspirations for them. Therefore, differences between the students' personal career choices and their parental aspirations are frequently a source of conflict.

Acculturation Status and Attitudes Toward Counseling and Therapy

Whether an Asian American seeks counseling for vocational issues or therapy for mental health issues, it is important to understand how such a person's background influences his/her attitude. Atikinson and Gim [94] inquired about how Asians view seeking professional help. Surveying 557 Chinese-, Japanese-, and Korean-American students, they found that the more highly acculturated students were more likely to recognize a personal need for professional psychological services. In addition, they were more open to discussing problems with a psychologist and were more tolerant of the stigma associated with psychological help. Given the stress confronting international students, Zhang [95] was also interested in their attitudes toward help-seeking, and thus studied 170 international students attending school within the United States. Zhang's results confirmed the relationship between acculturation level and attitudes; students with higher levels of acculturation showed more positive attitudes toward seeking psychological help.

Even when open to seeking professional help, it would be valuable to know whether Asian Americans have special preferences for the type of counselor or therapist they see. Atikson et al. [96] determined that Asian American undergraduates preferred counselors with attitudes and values similar to themselves. Lowe [97] uncovered even more specific information regarding preferential matching. From 103 Asian American undergraduates, she reported that a counselor with collectivistic characteristics was perceived as more cross-culturally competent than a counselor using an individualistic approach. Because this group had also scored higher on collectivism values than individualistic values, the results support the premise that matching is a relevant factor. Of great interest is the work of Kim and Atkinson [98], which involved Asian American and European American counselors who conducted a brief career counseling session with Asian Americans. These were undergraduates volunteering for a study on career counseling methods in which Asian American volunteer clients participated in one 50-min career counseling session led by a trained European American female counselor. Results indicated that participants with high Asian values evaluated Asian American counselors as more empathic and credible than participants with low adherence to Asian values. Those with low Asian values (or high Western acculturation) evaluated the European American counselors as more empathic than did the participants with high adherence to Asian values (low Western acculturation).

Whereas the prior research focused on matching, another series has studied the counselor's behavioral styles as an influence on preference. Directive versus nondirective approaches to counseling have been specifically examined in a series of research (see, for example, Exum and Lau, 99). Atkinson et al. [100] conducted studies in which Asian American students evaluated audiotapes of a simulated counseling session with an Asian American student client. There were four conditions. In one tape, the counselor is identified as Asian American using a directive counseling style; in a second tape, the counselor is identified as Asian American but is using a nondirective approach; in a third tape, the counselor is identified as European American and is using a directive counseling style; and in the fourth tape, the counselor is identified as European American and is using a nondirective counseling approach. In all tapes, the client is portrayed as an Asian American student conflicted about selecting a career that would not be acceptable to the client's parents. Results showed that Asian American participants evaluated the Asian American counselor as more credible and approachable than the European American counselor. Furthermore, the directive counseling approach was viewed more positively than the nondirective approach. More recently, Li and Kim [101] obtained Asian American college student evaluations of a counselor using either a directive or a nondirective style. The brief session was focused on career counseling. These Asian American participants rated the counselor using directive counseling strategy as more cross-culturally competent and empathic. The level of acculturation did not affect the evaluations.

Although these prior studies focus on the counselor characteristics, two reports examined how Asian participants viewed their roles in counseling interactions. Fowler and Parliament [102] and Yuen and Tinsley [103] reported that Asians expect to assume less responsibility or motivation during counseling, which dovetails with their expectation that the counselor be more direct and act as an expert. European Americans or European Canadians, on the other hand, expect to have a more active role during counseling and do not expect the counselor to provide all the solutions. In both studies, the Asian participants were lower in acculturation level, that is, were highly Asian culture identified. These studies would suggest that the determination of match between patient and clinician may be recommended to precede an initial evaluation to evaluate patient expectation and compatibility with the potential therapist's role.

Summary

Acculturation is defined in this chapter as a process that can occur when two or more cultures interact together. A variety of measurement approaches have been developed to assess this process including measures of behaviors, measures of values, or measures combining both behaviors and values. Numerous research studies have examined the relationship between acculturation and certain outcomes. Acculturation status has been found significantly associated with physical health and health-related behaviors, with mental health symptoms and distress, with family adjustment, with school performance, with career decision-making, and with the counseling/psychotherapy process. The relationship of acculturation to these outcomes provides substantial support for discussing, measuring, and understanding the acculturation process among Asian Americans as well as for the continuation of research about acculturation.

References

1. Redfield R, Linton R, and Herskovitz M. Memorandum on the study of acculturation. Am Anthropol 1936;38:149–152.
2. Leininger M. *Nursing and Anthropology: Two Worlds to Blend*, New York: John Wiley and Sons, 1970.
3. Berry J. Psychology of acculturation: under-standing individuals moving between cultures. In: Brislin R, ed. *Applied Cross-Cultural Psychology*. Newbury Park, CA: Sage, 1990: 232–253.
4. Suinn R. SL-ASIA: Suinn-Lew Asian Self-Identity Acculturation Scale. www.awong.com/~randy/dad/slasia.html 1994.
5. Berry J. Acculturation as varieties of adaptation. In: Padilla A, ed. *Acculturation: Theory, Models and New Findings*. Boulder, CO: Westview Press, 1980:9–25.
6. Berry J, Trimble J, and Olmedo E. Assessment of acculturation. In Lonner W, and Berry J. eds. *Field Methods in Cross-Cultural Research*. Beverly Hills, CA: Sage. 1986: 291–324.
7. Moyerman D and Forman B. Acculturation and adjustment: a meta-analytic study. Hisp J Behav Sci 1991;14:163–200.
8. Lee W. Becoming an American consumer: a Cross-cultural study of consumer acculturation among Taiwanese, Taiwanese in the Unites States and Americans. Communications. Urbana-Champaign: University of Illinois, 1988.
9. Suinn R, Rickard-Figueroa K, Lew S, and Vigil P. The Suinn-Lew Asian Self-Identity Acculturation Scale: An Initial Report. Educ Psychol Meas 1987;47:402–407.
10. Suinn R, Ahuna C., and Khoo G. The Suinn-Lew Asian Self-Identity Acculturation Scale: concurrent and factorial validation. Educ Psychol Meas 1992;52:1041–1046.

11. Abe-Kim J, Okazaki S, and Goto S. Unidimensional versus multidimensional approaches to the assessment of acculturation for Asian American populations. *Cultur Divers Ethnic Minor Psychol* 2001;7:232–246.
12. Mallinckrodt B, Shigeoka S, and Suzuki L. Asian and Pacific Island American students' acculturation and etiology beliefs about typical counseling presenting problems. Cultur Divers Ethnic Minor Psychol 2005;11:227–238.
13. Chung R, Kim B, and Abreu, J. Asian American Multidimensional Acculturation Scale: development, factor analysis, reliability and validity. Cultur Divers Ethnic Minor Psychol 2004;10:66–80.
14. Kim B. Acculturation and enculturation. In: Leong F, Inman A. Ebreo A, Yang L, Kinoshita L, and Fu M. eds. *Handbook of Asian-American Psychology*, 2nd edn. Thousand Oaks, CA: Sage, 2006:141–158.
15. Leong F. The role of acculturation in the career adjustment of Asian American workers: a test of Leong and Chou's (1994) formulations. *Cult Diver Ethnic Minor Psychol* 2001;7:262–273.
16. Johnson M, Wall T, Guanipa C, Terry-Guyer L, and Velasquez R. The psychometric properties of the Orthogonal Cultural Identification Scale in Asian Americans. *J Multicult Couns Dev* 2002;30:181–190.
17. Gupta R and Yick A. Preliminary validation of the acculturation scale on Chinese Americans. *J Soc Work Res Eval* 2001;1 2:43–56.
18. Marin G, Sabogal F, Marin B, Otero-Sabogal R, and Perez-Stable E. Development of a short acculturation scale for Hispanics. *Hisp J Behav Sci* 1987;9:183–205
19. Kim B, Atkinson D, and Yang P. The Asian values scale: development, factor analysis, validation, and reliability. *J Couns Psychol* 1999;46:342–352.
20. Kim B and Hong S. A psychometric revision of the Asian values scale using the Rasch model. *Meas Eval Counsel Dev* 2004; 37:15–27.
21. Kim B, Li L, and Ng F. The Asian American values scale-multidimensional: development, reliability, and validity. *Cultur Divers Ethnic Minor Psychol* 2005;11: 187–201
22. Wolfe M, Yang P, Wong E, and Atkinson D. Design and development of the European American values scale for Asian Americans. *Cultur Divers Ethnic Minor Psychol* 2001;7: 274–283.
23. Hong S, Kim B, and Wolf, M. A psychometric revision of the European American values scale for Asian Americans using the Rasch model. *Meas Eval Counsel Dev* 2005;37: 194–207.
24. Nguyen H and von Eye A. The acculturation scale for Vietnamese adolescents (ASVA): a bidimensional perspective. *Int J Behav Dev* 2002;26: 202–213.
25. Stephenson M. Development and validation of the Stephenson Multigroup Acculturation Scale (SMAS). *Psychol Assess* 2000;12:77–88.
26. Unger J, Gallaher P, Shakib S, Ritt-Olson A, Palmer P, and Johnson C. AHIMSA acculturation scale: a new measure of acculturation for adolescents in a multicultural society. *J Early Adolesc* 2002;22:225–251.
27. Wong-Rieger D and Quintana D. Comparative acculturation of Southeast Asian and Hispanic immigrants and sojourners. *J Cross Cult Psychol* 1987;18:345–362.
28. Oetting E and Beauvais F. Orthogonal cultural identification theory: the cultural identification of minority adolescents. *Int J Addict* 1990–1991;25;655–685.
29. Venner K, Wall T, Lau P, and Ehlers C. (2006). Testing of an orthogonal measure of cultural identification with adult mission Indians. *Cultur Divers Ethnic Minor Psychol* 2006;4:632–643.
30. Marmot M, Syme S, Kagan A, Kato H, Cohen J, and Belsky J. Epidemiologic studies of coronary heart disease and stroke in Japanese men living in Japan, Hawaii and California: prevalence of coronary and hypertensive heart disease and associated risk factors. *Am J Epidemiol* 1975;102:514–25.
31. Robertson T, Kato H, Rhoads G, Kagan A, Marmot M, Syme S, Gordon T, Worth R, Belsky J, Dock D, Miyanishi M, and Kawamoto S. Epidemiologic studies of coronary

heart disease and stroke in Japanese men living in Japan, Hawaii and California. Incidence of myocardial infarction and death from coronary heart disease. *Am J Cardiol* 1977;39:239–43.
32. Kaplan M, Chang C, Newsom J, and McFarland B. Acculturation status and hypertension among Asian immigrants in Canada. *J Epidemol Community Health* 2002;56:455–456.
33. Mau S. The relationship of eating attitudes, body image preferences, and *acculturation* on adolescent girls in Hong Kong. *Diss Abstr: Sect B: Sci Eng* 2000;60(8-B), Mar. :4235.
34. Garner D, Olmsted M, Bohr Y, and Garfinkel P. The eating attitudes test: psychometric features and clinical correlates. *Psychol Med* 1982;12:871–878.
35. Garner D, Olmstead M, and Polivy J. Development and validation of a multidimensional Eating Disorder Inventory for anorexia nervosa and bulimia. *Int J Eat Disord* 1983;2: 15–34.
36. Doan L. Eating disorder symptomatology, East *Asian* culture, and modes of acculturation. *Diss Abstr Sect B:Sci Eng* 2001; 62(1-B), July: 544.
37. Stark-Wroblewski K, Yanico B, and Lupe S. Acculturation, internalization of western appearance norms, and eating pathology among Japanese and Chinese international student women. *Psychol Women Q* 2005;29:38–46.
38. Unger J, Reynolds K, Shakip S, Spruijt-Metz D, Sun P, and Johnson C. Acculturation, physical activity, and fast-food consumption among Asian-American and Hispanic adolescents. *J Community Health* 2004;29:467–481.
39. Yang J. The relationship between contextual factors of psychological distress with emotional eating and body weight in Hmong and Hmong American college populations. Doctoral dissertation, Alliant University: Fresno, CA, 2006.
40. Ma G, Tan Y, Toubehh J, and Su X. Differences in stages of change of smoking behavior among current smokers of four Asian American subgroups. *Addict Behav* 2003;28: 1431–1439.
41. Unger J, Trinidad D, Weiss J, and Rohrbach L. Acculturation as a risk factor for smoking among Asian American adolescents: is the Association Confounded by Nationality? *J Ethn Subst Abuse* 2004;3:65–79.
42. Ma G, Tan Y, Toubbeh J, Su X, Shive S, and Lan Y. Acculturation and smoking behavior in Asian-American populations. *Health Educ Res* 2004;19: 615–625.
43. Hofstetter C, Hovell M, Lee J, Zakarian J, Park H, Paik H, and Irvin V. Tobacco use and acculturation among Californians of Korean descent: a behavioral epidemiological analysis. *Nicotine Tob Res* 2004;6:481–489.
44. Weiss J and Garbanati J. Relationship of acculturation and family functioning to smoking attitudes and behaviors among Asian-American adolescents. *J Child Fam Stud* 2004;13:193–204.
45. Chen X, Unger J, Cruz T, and Johnson C. Smoking patterns of Asian-American youth in California and their relationship with acculturation. *J Adolesc Health* 1999;24:321–328.
46. Unger J, Cruz T, Rohrbach L, Ribisi K, Baezconde-Garbanati L, Chen X, Trinidad, D, and Johnson C. English language use as a risk actor for smoking initiation among Hispanic and Asian American adolescents: evidence for mediation by tobacco-related believes and social norms. *Health Psychol* 2000; 19:403–410.
47. Unger J and Chen X. The role of social networks and media receptivity in predicting age of smoking initiation: a proportional hazards model of risk and protective factors. *Addict Behav* 1999;24:371–381.
48. Unger J, Yan, L, Shaki, S, Rohrbach L, Chen X, Qian G, Chou C, Jianguo S, Azen S, Zheng H, and Johnson C. Peer influences and access to cigarettes as correlates of adolescent smoking: a cross-cultural comparison of Wuhan, China and California. *Prev Med*; 2002;34:476–484.
49. Hahm H, Lahiff M, and Guterman N. Acculturation and parental attachment in Asian-American adolescents' alcohol use. *J Adolesc Health* 2003;33:119–129.

50. Hendershot C, MacPherson, L, Myers M, Carr L, and Wall T. Psychosocial, cultural and genetic influences on alcohol use in Asian American Youth. *J Stud Alcohol* 2005;66: 185–195.
51. Hahm H, Lahiff M, and Guterman N. Asian American adolescents' acculturation, binge drinking, and alcohol- and tobacco-using peers. *J Community Psychol* 2004;32:295–308.
52. Berry, J. Marginality, stress and ethnic identification in an acculturated aboriginal community. *J Cross-Cult Psychol* 1970;1:239–252.
53. Berry J, Kim U, Minde T, and Mok D. Comparative studies of acculturative stress. *Int Migr Rev* 1987;21:491–511.
54. Liang C, Li L, and Kim B. The Asian American racism-related stress inventory: development, factor analysis, reliability, and validity. *J Counsel Psychol* 2004;51:103–114.
55. Mays V, Cochran S, and Barnes N. Race, race-based discrimination, and health outcomes among African Americans. *Annu Rev Psychol* 2007;58:201–225.
56. Mio J, Nagata D, Tsai A, and Tweari N. Racism against Asian/Pacific Americans. In: Leong F, Inman A, Ebreo A, Yan L. Kinoshita L, and Fu M. eds. *Handbook of Asian-American Psychology*, 2nd edn. Sage Publications, Thousand Oaks, CA 2006:341–461.
57. Sue D, Bucceri J, Lin A, Nadal K, and Torino G. Racial microaggressions and the Asian American experience. *Cultur Divers Ethnic Minor Psychol* 2007;13:72–81.
58. Sodowsky G and Lai E. Asian immigrant variables and structural models of cross-cultural distdress. In: Booth A. ed. *International Migration and Family Change: The Exeprience of U.S. Immigrants* . Mahwah, N.J. Erblaum, 1997: 211–237.
59. Wang C and Mallinckrodt B. Acculturation, attachment, and psychosocial adjustment of Chinese/Taiwanese International students. *Cultur Divers Ethnic Minor Psychol* 2006;53:422–433.
60. Wilton L and Constantine M. Length of residence, cultural adjustment difficulties, and psychological distress symptoms in Asian and Latin American international college students. *J Coll Counsel* 2003:6:177–187.
61. Lee J, Koeske G, and Sales E. Social support buffering of acculturative stress: a study of mental health symptoms among Korean international students. *Int J Intercult Rel* 2004:28:399–414.
62. Ryder A, Alden L, and Paulhus D Is acculturation unidimensional or bidimensional? *J Pers Soc Psychol* 2000;79:49–65.
63. Chung R, Bemak F, and Wong S. Social support and acculturation: implications for mental health counseling. *J Ment Health Couns* 2000;22:150–161.
64. Shen B and Takeuchi D. A structural model of acculturation and mental health status among Chinese Americans. *Am J Community Psychol* 2001;29:387–418.
65. Kim S, Gonzales N, Stroh, and Wang J. Parent-child cultural marginalization and depressive symptoms in Asian American family members. *J Community Psychol* 2006;34:167–182
66. Crane D, Ngal S, Larson J, and Hafen M. The influence of family functioning and parent–adolescent acculturation on North American Chinese adolescent outcomes. *Fam Relat* 2005;54:400–410.
67. Lau A, Jernewall N, Zane N, and Myers H. Correlates of suicidal behaviors among Asian American outpatient youths. *Cultur Divers Ethnic Minor Psychol* 2002;8:199–213.
68. Fu M. Acculturation, ethnic identity, and *family conflict* among first- and second-generation Chinese Americans. *Diss Abstr: Sect B: Sci Eng* 2002;63(2-B), Aug.:1024.
69. Nguyen, G. The relationship between differential acculturation levels, family conflct , and self-esteem among Vietnamese-Americans. *Diss Abstr: Sect B: Sci Eng* 2003;64 (4-B):1943.
70. Pyke K. "Generational Deserters" and "Black Sheep": acculturative differences among siblings in Asian immigrant families. *J Fam Issues* 2005;26:491–517.
71. Sharir I. Chinese immigrant youth in Vancouver, Canada: an examination of acculturation, adjustment, and intergenerational conflict. *Diss Abstr: Sect B: Sci Eng*. 2002;63 (4-B), Oct.:2075.

72. Ying Y and Han M. The longitudinal effect of intergenerational gap in acculturation on conflict and mental health in Southeast Asian American adolescents. *Am J Orthopsychiatry* 2007;77: 61–66.
73. Kim U and Chun M. Educational 'success' of Asian Americans: an indigenous perspective. *J Appl Dev Psychol* 1994;15:329–339.
74. Sue S and Okazaki S. Asian-American educational achievements: a phenomenon in search of an explanation. *Am Psychol* 1990;45:913–920.
75. Huntsinger C, Jose P, Larson S, Krieg D, and Shaligram C. Mathematics, vocabulary, and reading development in Chinese American and European American Children Over the Primary School Years. *J Educ Psychol* 2000;92:745–760.
76. Fuligini A, Witkow M., and Garcia C. Ethnic identity and the academic adjustment of adolescents from Mexican, Chinese, and European Backgrounds. *Dev Psychol* 2005;41: 799–811.
77. Dandy J and Nettelbeck T. A cross-cultural study of parents' *academic* standards and educational aspirations for their children. *Educ Psychol* 2002;22:621–627.
78. Pringle C and Rasinski K. The National Education Longitudinal Study of 1988: Data Collection Results and Analysis Potential. Paper presented at the Annual Meeting of the American Educational Research Association, San Francisco, California, March 27, 1989. Also available as NELS:88 report ED 295 985, ED308215, TM013551, RIEN0V89.
79. Shin H. Parental involvement and its influence on children's school performance: a comparative study between Asian (Chinese and Koreans) Americans and Mexican-Americans. Unpublished Doctoral dissertation. Columbia University, 2004.
80. Goyette K and Xie Y. Educational expectations of Asian American youths: determinants and *ethnic differences. Sociol Educ* 1999;72:22–36.
81. Peng S and Wright D. Explanation of *academic achievement* of Asian American *students*. *J Educ Res* 1994;87:346–352
82. Mizokawa D and Ryckman D. Attributions of *academic* success and failure: a comparison of six Asian-American ethnic groups. *J Cross Cult Psychol* 1990;21:434–451.
83. Hau K and Salili F. Structure and semantic differential placement of specific causes: *Academic* causal attributions by Chinese *students* in Hong Kong. *Int J Psychol* 1991;26: 175–193.
84. Yan W and Gaien E. Causal *attributions* for college *success* and failure: an American - Asian comparison. *J Cross Cult Psychol* 1994;25:146–158.
85. Chao R. Beyond parental control and authoritarian parenting style: understanding Chinese parenting through the cultural notion of training. *Child Dev* 1994;65: 111–1119.
86. Chalip L and Stigler J. The development of achievement and ability among Chinese children: a new contribution to an old controversy. *J Educ Res* 1986;79:302–307.
87. Stevenson H, Lee S, and Stigler J. Mathematics achievement of Chinese, Japanese and American children. Science 1986;231:693–699.
88. Wu D. Chinese childhood socialization. In Bond M. ed. The Handbook of Chinese Psychology. Hong Kong: Oxford University Press 1996:143–154.
89. Tang M, Fouad N, and Smith P. Asian Americans career choices: a path model to examine the factors influencing choices. *J Vocat Behav* 1999;54:142–157.
90. Castelino P. Factors influencing career choices of South Asian Americans: a path analysis. *Diss Abstr* 2005. *Sect A: Humanit Soc Sci* 65 (8-A):2906.
91. Hsieh M. Sociocultural factors influencing career indecision of Asian/Asian-American female college students: a cross-cultural comparison. *Diss Abstr. Sect A: Humanit Soc Sci*, 1996; 56(11-A):4325.
92. Tang M. A comparison of Asian American, Caucasian American, and Chinese college students: an initial report. *J Multicult Couns Dev* 2002;30:124–134.
93. Corey A. Correlates of Asian American college students' career aspirations: generational status, self-reports, and parental-reports on *acculturation* and perceived prejudice. *Diss Abstr.Sect B: Sci Eng*, 2001;61(7-B), Feb:3837.

94. Atkinson D and Gim R. Asian-American cultural identity and attitudes toward mental health services. *J Couns Psychol* 1989;36:209–212.
95. Zhang N. Acculturation and counseling expectancies: Asian international students' attitudes toward seeking professional psychological help. (Asian students). *Diss Abstr Sect A: Humanit Soc Sci*, 2000;60(7-A), Jan.:2392.
96. Atkinson D, Wampold B, Lowe S, Matthews L, and Ahn H. Asian American preferences for counselor characteristics: application of the Bradley–Terry–Luce model to paired comparison data. *Couns Psychol* 1998;26:101–123.
97. Lowe S. Impact of individualist and collectivist approaches to career counseling with Asian-Americans on perceptions of counselor cross-cultural competence and credibility. *Diss Abstr Sect A: Humanit Soc Sci*, 1999;60(2-A:0348.
98. Kim B and Atkinson D. Effects of Asian American client adherence to Asian cultural values, counselor expression of cultural values, and counselor ethnicity on career counseling process. *J Couns Psychol* 2002;49:3–13.
99. Exum H and Lau E. Counseling style preference of Chinese college students. *J Multicult Couns Dev* 1988;16:84–92.
100. Atkinson D, Maruyama M, and Matsui, S. Effects of counselor race and counseling approach on Asian Americans' perceptions of counselor credibility and utility. *J Couns Psychol* 1978;25:76–283.
101. Li L and Kim B. Effects of counseling style and client adherence to Asian cultural values on counseling process with Asian American college students. *J Couns Psychol* 2004;51: 158–167.
102. Fowler D and Parliament V. The influence of culture on therapeutic expectations. Unpublished undergraduate thesis. Halifax, Nova Scotia: St. Mary's University 2005.
103. Yuen R and Tinsley H. International and American students' expectations about counseling. *J Couns Psychol* 1981;28:66–69.

Theories and Research on Acculturation and Enculturation Experiences among Asian American Families

Bryan S. K. Kim, Annie J. Ahn, and N. Alexandra Lam

Abstract In this chapter, we define and discuss the concepts of acculturation and enculturation, as well as theories and research on the consequences of acculturation and enculturation for Asian American families. We also explore the roles acculturation and enculturation play on parent–child values gap and family conflict, the role of cognitive flexibility in this relationship, and clinical implications of the findings.

Keywords Acculturation · Enculturation · Cultural values · Asian American families · Family conflict

Contents

Construct Definitions of Acculturation and Enculturation for Asian American Families	26
Theories and Research on the Consequences of Acculturation and Enculturation for Asian American Families	28
Relationships among Parent–Child Cultural Values Gap, Cognitive Flexibility, and Family Conflict	32
Method	33
Instruments	33
Results	36
Preliminary Analysis	36
Main Analyses	37
Discussion of the Results	38
Limitations and Implications	40
Conclusion	41
References	41

Asian American families comprise units with diverse immigration histories. For example, many of these families are five and six generations removed from

B.S.K. Kim
Department of Psychology, University of Hawaii at Hilo, Hilo, HI 96720-4091, USA
e-mail: bryankim@hawaii.edu

migration, whose ancestors entered the United States in the mid-1800s and early 1900s during the sugar and pineapple plantation period in Hawaii and the Gold Rush and Transcontinental Railroad eras in California. Other families are third- and fourth-generation Americans whose Asian ancestors entered the United States during World War II and the Korean War. There are also Asian American families who entered the United States after the passing of the Immigration Act of 1965 or after the United States' pullout from Southeast Asia in 1975. Moreover, Asian American families comprise members who entered the United States as recently as yesterday. This suggests that Asian Americans represent a wide range of diversity to the extent to which they have adopted the norms of the dominant US culture and retained the norms of the traditional Asian culture.

To understand this type of diversity among Asian American families, the constructs of acculturation and enculturation can be very useful. Therefore, in this chapter, we will describe the definitions of these two concepts and explore related psychological theories and research with Asian American families. These sections will be followed by a description of a recently completed research study that examined the role of *values enculturation* in the conflicts experienced between parents and children. Specifically, the study examined the cultural values gap between Asian American parents and their children and its relations to respondents' cognitive flexibility and conflicts within the family.

Construct Definitions of Acculturation and Enculturation for Asian American Families

Acculturation was first defined by Redfield et al. (1936) [1] as follows: "Acculturation comprehends those phenomena which result when groups of individuals sharing different cultures come into continuous first-hand contact, with subsequent changes in the original culture patterns of either or both groups" (p. 149).

Several decades later, Graves (1967) [2] used the term *psychological acculturation* to describe the effects of acculturation at the individual level. This process involves changes that an individual experiences in terms of their attitudes, values, and identity as a result of being in contact with other cultures. John Berry and his colleagues [3, 4] developed a bilinear model of acculturation in which one linearity represented "*contact and participation* (to what extent should they become involved in other cultural groups, or remain primarily among themselves)" and the other linearity represented "*cultural maintenance* (to what extent are cultural identity and characteristics considered to be important, and their maintenance striven for)" (p. 304, 305).

Closely related to the construct of acculturation is the concept of *enculturation*. First defined by Herskovits (1948) [5], enculturation refers to the process of socialization into and maintenance of the norms of one's indigenous culture, including its salient ideas, concepts, and values. Recently, BSK Kim (2007) [6] pointed out that the "cultural maintenance" process that is described above might be better represented with the broader terminology of enculturation.

Although the above characterization of cultural maintenance may accurately describe the experiences of Asian American migrants who already had been socialized into their traditional Asian cultural norms before entering the United States, it may not be accurate for Asian Americans who are one or more generations removed from migration. For these individuals who were born in the United States, they may never have been fully enculturated into their Asian ethnic group's cultural norms and may not be engaged in the process of cultural maintenance. Hence, for these individuals, the use of the term cultural maintenance may be inappropriate. Rather, the concept of enculturation provides a more comprehensive description of socialization into and maintenance of one's indigenous cultural norms. Furthermore, BSK Kim (2007) [6] pointed out that an additional benefit of using the term enculturation is that it places an equal level of focus on the process of learning and retaining one's Asian cultural norms as acculturation, which has largely focused on the process of adapting to the norms of the US culture.

Consistent with this explanation, BSK Kim and Abreu (2001) [7] proposed that enculturation be used to describe the process of (re)learning and maintaining the norms of the indigenous culture, and acculturation be used to describe the process of adapting to the norms of the dominant culture. For Asian American families, therefore, acculturation refers to the process of adapting to the norms of the US culture, and enculturation refers to the process of becoming socialized into and maintaining the norms of the Asian culture. Current understanding of acculturation and enculturation suggests that Asian American families who are further removed from immigration will be more acculturated and therefore adhere to the mainstream US norms more strongly than Asian American families who are recent migrants [8]. On the other hand, Asian Americans who are closer to migration will be more enculturated and therefore adhere to Asian norms more strongly than their counterparts who are one or more generations removed from immigration.

In studying acculturation and enculturation, it is also important to consider the construct dimensions on which the two types of adherence can be observed and assessed. Szapocznik et al. (1978) [9] first elaborated on the ways of assessing acculturation (and enculturation) by proposing that it involves changes in behaviors and values. According to these authors, the behavioral dimension of acculturation includes language use and participation in various cultural activities (e.g., food consumption), whereas the values dimension reflects relational style, person–nature relationships, beliefs about human nature, and time orientation (e.g., present-focused, future-focused, or past-focused).

More recently, BSK Kim and Abreu (2001) [7] reviewed the items in 33 instruments designed to measure acculturation and enculturation and, based on their finding, proposed that acculturation and enculturation constructs encompass four dimensions. These authors proposed the following dimensions: *behavior*, *values*, *knowledge*, and *identity*. Behavior refers to friendship choice, preferences for television program and reading, participation in cultural activities, contact with indigenous culture (e.g., time spent in the country of origin), language use, food choice, and music preference. The value dimension refers to attitudes and beliefs about social relations, cultural customs, and cultural traditions, in addition gender roles and attitudes and ideas about health and illness. The knowledge dimension refers to culturally specific information such as names of historical leaders in the culture of origin and the dominant culture, and significance of culturally specific activities. The cultural identity dimension refers to attitudes toward one's cultural identification (e.g., preferred name is in Korean), attitudes toward indigenous and dominant groups (e.g., feelings of pride toward the indigenous group), and the level of comfort toward the people of indigenous and dominant groups. In classifying identity as one of these four dimensions, BSK Kim and Abreu (2001) [7] pointed out that this concept largely overlaps with the construct of ethnic and racial identity; indeed, "acculturation" and "ethnic and racial identity" are constructs that are not well differentiated in the literature [10]. Also, BSK Kim and Abreu (2001) [7] pointed out that the four dimensions of acculturation and enculturation are not unrelated to each other. For example, the behavioral and knowledge dimensions may be correlated, as behavior is likely to be preceded by knowledge, a principle that also applies to other pairs of dimensions.

Theories and Research on the Consequences of Acculturation and Enculturation for Asian American Families

To understand the acculturation and enculturation experiences of Asian American families in the context of mental health, an important area to explore is the potential consequences of differential rates of progress between parents and children along both acculturation and enculturation continua. Therefore, in this section, the current theories and research on the potential consequences of differential rates of acculturation and enculturation will be described.

To further expound on the concept of "conflict," Hwang (2007) [11] proposed the term Acculturative Family Distancing (AFD) to describe the family functioning among Asian Americans with respect to varying levels of acculturation and enculturation between parents and children. Specifically, AFD is defined as "the problematic distancing that occurs between immigrant parents and children that is a consequence of differences in acculturative [and enculturative] processes and cultural changes that become more salient over time" (p. 398, 11). AFD consists of two dimensions: "a breakdown in communication and incongruent cultural values that develop as a consequence of different rates of acculturation and the formation of an acculturation gap" (p. 398, 11). Hwang (2007) [11] posited that AFD increases the development of problems through distancing in the realms of emotion, cognition, and behavior, which eventually lead to family conflict. In our research study described below, the dimension of incongruent cultural values was explored in terms of its relation to family conflicts, as well as the possible moderating role of cognitive flexibility in this relation. In this chapter, cognitive flexibility refers to an individual's awareness that, in any situation, there are options and alternatives available, willingness to be flexible and adapt to the situation, and self-efficacy in being flexible.

Similar to AFD, Rosenthal et al. (1989) [12] described how parent–child conflicts occur through a "culture conflict model." This model proposed that although parents tend to cling to the values from their culture of origin to gain a sense of control over adjusting to an unfamiliar culture, children might increasingly adopt the norms of the dominant society. Because children arrive to the United States at an earlier age, they have more experiences with its cultural norms such as through school, media, and interactions with peers than their parents [13, 14]. During the process of being exposed to two cultures, problems can surface between parents and children when the norms of the culture of origin are vastly different from those of the dominant culture [15, 16]. This dynamic also has been labeled as "dissonant acculturation" [17].

Ryu and Vann (1992) [18] provided a conceptual description of how conflicts can occur between Asian American parents and children. Already feeling a loss of power over their personal life from immigration-related stressors, Asian American parents, when their authority is also threatened, may demand unconditional obedience from their children. For example, parents may overemphasize the importance of excellent grades and view academic achievement as the only way to be successful in the United States. In turn, children may become overwhelmed by these pressures, as they are also attempting to fit in with their peers from the dominant culture, form their own ethnic identity, and try to show genuine respect for their parents' wishes [19]. Consequently, children may experience a type of double bind where they feel rejected from both their Asian culture and the host culture [20]. Parents may feel betrayed by their children who appear to be resistant to their influencing efforts [21, 20].

JM Kim (2003) [23] described how conflicts can develop from the contrasting emphases of traditional Asian values and values from the dominant culture and differential rates of children's and parent's acculturation in Asian American families. Asian cultural values emphasize interdependence and filial piety, which are in direct opposition to American values that emphasize independence. When children adapt more to American values and parents choose to adhere more to Asian values, parents often feel bewildered and overwhelmed as they interpret their children's rejection of traditional values personally. Fearing the loss of control over their children, parents may get anxious and commonly view children's behaviors as selfish or indifferent to their family ties. On the other hand, children may feel frustrated, angry, and rebellious toward their parents' lack of acceptance of their growing self-assertions and self-reliance.

LaFromboise et al. (1993) [24] also pointed out that immigrant families in particular are vulnerable to psychological distress because of their adjustment with the opposing demands of two cultures. Referred to as *acculturative stress*, problems can occur when Asian American families have trouble adjusting to the US norms while trying to retain the norms of their indigenous culture. These problems can lead to symptoms such as worsened mental health status, anxiety, depression, feelings of marginality and alienation, identity confusion, and psychosomatic symptoms [25]. But on the more positive side, these authors also pointed out that once individuals have achieved biculturalism, where individuals are able to function well within the norms of both cultures, positive benefits can be experienced. In support of this idea, a study with Vietnamese youths living in a primarily European American community explored possible links between their acculturation process and adjustment [26]. The results showed that the youths who were strongly involved with both American and Vietnamese cultures tended to have more positive family relationships and higher self-esteem. But youths who were involved only in Vietnamese culture and not with the predominant European American culture experienced more psychological distress. Collectively, these results suggest that there are strong benefits to achieving biculturalism with both the dominant and indigenous cultures.

Within the framework of bicultural competence is cognitive flexibility, a construct that could serve as a helpful buffer against psychological distress arising from acculturation and enculturation processes. As mentioned earlier, cognitive flexibility refers to the awareness that in any situation there are options and alternatives available, the willingness to be flexible and adapt to the situation, and the competence to be flexible [27]. It represents the ability of bicultural individuals to cope with and reconcile potential conflicts as they try to function in two different cultural norms. Harrison et al. (1990) [28] observed that increased cognitive flexibility is one of the benefits experienced by children who grow up in ethnic minority families in the United States in which the children learn to negotiate the demands of the two cultures. Related to this observation, a study by Ahn et al. (2005) [29] found that increased cognitive flexibility was related to decreased likelihood and seriousness of child–parent conflicts among Korean Americans, particularly in the area of children's education and career. In the study described in the second half of this chapter, cognitive flexibility is examined as a possible moderator on the relation between parent–child cultural values gap and family conflict.

In addition to these internal family dynamics between immigrant parents and children, Asian American families in general also experience environmental and sociopolitical stressors that can exacerbate the parent–child conflicts that occur at home. Particularly, the experience of racism due to their minority status can cause stress for each family member and negatively impact the family dynamics [30, 31]. More specifically, Chan and Hune (1995) [32] explained that the needs of the Asian American group tend to be ignored by policy makers and institutional leaders. Instead, Asian Americans are often scapegoated during times of economic recession and social crisis. Asian Americans are subject to stereotypes and are excluded from school curricula, media representation, and popular culture. Furthermore, Asian Americans are at risk of the glass ceiling effect, receiving lower wages than European Americans who have equal or lower training and education. Moreover, there exist anti-immigrant sentiment, anti-Asian violence, and occupational segregations that increase the risk of psychological stress among Asian American families. These risk factors in turn can make it even more difficult for parents and children to cope with conflicts that may exist between them.

There have been a growing number of research studies focusing on the acculturation and enculturation experiences of Asian American families. In one of the first studies on this topic, Wakil et al. (1981) [33] found that Asian American parents might be open to adopting pragmatic aspects of the dominant culture. For example, the participants tended to relinquish some of the traditional Asian gender norms and encourage their daughters to obtain professional degrees. The parents tended to allow their children to have more choices in their education and occupational decisions. To explain these findings, the author(s) pointed out that the parents viewed these changes as "functional compromises," which allowed them to remain strongly embedded in traditional core values such as the importance of family influence on selecting a marriage partner.

In a related study, Nguyen and William (1989) [34] found that Asian American parents might send mixed messages with regard to which traditional values to endorse. The study involved Vietnamese and European American adolescents from 12 to 19 years old in the Oklahoma City public schools and their parents. The participants completed a questionnaire assessing family values, which included Vietnamese values and issues of adolescent independence. The study revealed that Vietnamese parents strongly endorsed family values and absolute obedience to authority but that the adolescents rejected these traditional values. Interestingly, the results also showed that parents were ambivalent about giving children rights and privileges in their dating, marriage, and career choices.

A few studies have pointed to gender as an important factor leading to an increase in the levels of parent–child conflict. Particularly, females reported more conflict compared with males in areas of gender role expectations and dating and marriage issues [34–36]. In support of these earlier results, Chung (2001) [19] found that male students reported a lower number of conflicts with their parents regarding dating and marriage issues in comparison with their female counterparts.

In terms of the specific content areas of disagreement between Asian American parents and children, a study by Kwak and Berry (2001) [37] revealed that in comparison with European Americans, Asian Americans experienced more parent–child disagreements in the areas of independence, roles in decision-making, and intercultural contact. Asian American parents tended to view parental authority and children's rights from the perspective of their culture of origin, whereas adolescents tended to adopt more to the independent values of dominant US culture. In addition, Lowinger and Kwok (2001) [38] found that Asian American parents tend to engage in parental overprotection. Parental overprotection refers to the stifling of a child's emotional autonomy and independence, as well as nonresponsiveness to the child's needs for acceptance and approval. Studies have found that parental overprotection can lead to deleterious effects for Asian American children growing up in Western societies [21, 39]. For example, research suggests that parent overprotection in the form of parental strictness can be interpreted as a sign of hostility, aggression, distrust, and rejection, which can lead to a decrease in children's self-confidence and assertiveness, children doubting their parents' love, and decreased ability for children to be extroverted. Moreover, children who experience academic pressure from their parents without support and praise for their accomplishments may become anxious, obsessive-compulsive, and depressed [38].

In a recent study, Ahn et al. (2005) [29] directly investigated the role of enculturation on the occurrence of parent–child conflicts among Korean Americans. These authors examined Korean American college students' perceived Asian cultural values gap between themselves and their parents, their cognitive flexibility, and their coping strategies. The relationships between these factors were studied, which included the intensities and types of child–parent conflicts. The results indicated that the students generally adhered less strongly to Asian values than their parents. When faced with conflicts, the respondents reported using a problem-solving coping strategy to the greatest extent, followed by a social support coping strategy, and then an avoidance coping strategy. There was a positive relationship between the student-perceived student–parent values gap and the intensity of conflicts, particularly in the area of dating and marriage. In contrast, there were inverse relationships between cognitive flexibility and the intensity of conflicts, specifically in the area of dating and marriage. Furthermore, a positive relationship was observed between the intensity level of conflicts and the use of social support coping strategy. Surprisingly, there was an interaction effect where student-perceived student–parent values gap and cognitive flexibility were related to increased frequency of conflicts around the topic of whom the child should date or marry. However, an important limitation of this study was that parents' cultural values orientation was based on the perceptions of the student and not directly from the parents themselves.

To summarize, current theory and research findings suggest that many Asian American parents and children have differences in world views, and these differences can lead to parent–child conflicts and other negative psychological outcomes. One area in which these differences manifest themselves is that Asian American parents tend to hold onto the traditional Asian values more tightly than their children. Asian American children, given their increased exposure to dominant US cultural norms, tend to more readily relinquish traditional Asian values and adhere to the values of the dominant US culture. In essence, there are differential rates of enculturation and acculturation between Asian American parents and their children.

Relationships among Parent–Child Cultural Values Gap, Cognitive Flexibility, and Family Conflict

This study represented an extension of the study of Ahn et al. (2005) [29], in that the relationship between child–parent cultural values gap and intergenerational conflict was explored using actual reports from both parents and children, rather than the perceived values gap by the children as was done in Ahn et al. (2005) [29]. Specifically, we examined the actual child–parent Asian values gap and its possible relation to child-perceived conflicts. In addition, the child's cognitive flexibility was examined as a possible moderator on this relation.

Method

Participants

The participants were 146 Korean American parent–child dyads. The children were college students who attended one of the four large West Coast Universities or two West Coast Korean churches. The child sample consisted of 80 females and 66 males and their ages ranged from 17 to 33 years ($M = 20.62$, $SD = 2.18$). There were 46 seniors (31.5%), 34 sophomores (23.3%), 33 juniors (22.6%), 22 freshmen (15.1%); 6 graduate students (4.1%), and 5 did not report grade level. There were 41 (28.1%) first-generation and 101 (69.2%) second-generation students, and 4 did not report their generation status. Among the first-generation students, the mean number of years in the United States was 12.48 years ($SD = 4.84$) with a range of 2 months to 22 years. At the time of data collection, 55 (37.7%) students reported living with their parents, whereas 90 (61.6%) reported living away from their parents; 1 did not report his or her living status.

The parent sample consisted of 96 mothers and 50 fathers, whose ages ranged from 42 to 64 years ($M = 50.42$, $SD = 4.14$). Of these, 127 parents (87%) completed the Korean version of the survey and 19 (13%) completed the English version of the questionnaire. Overall 87% of parents were foreign born with an average length of stay of 22.65 years in the United States ($SD = 8.69$) with a range of 5–61 years. In terms of marital status, 112 (76.7%) parents were married, 23 (15.8%) were divorced, 3 (2.1%) were separated, 5 (3.4%) were widowed, and 2 (1.4%) were single; 1 did not respond. In terms of the educational background of mothers, there were 7 (4.8%) with less than a high school degree, 51(34.9%) high school degree, 62 (42.5%) bachelor of arts degree, 13 (8.9%) masters degree, 1 (0.7%) MBA, 2 (1.4%) Ph.D., and 10 (6.8%) reported other. The fathers' educational background consisted of 4 (2.8%) with less than a high school degree, 32 (22.4%) high school degree, 60 (42.0%) bachelor of arts degree, 18 (12.6%) masters degree, 6 (4.2%) MBA, 9 (6.3%) Ph.D., 11 (7.7%) listed other, and 6 did not report.

Instruments

To assess the variables examined in this study, we utilized the following instrument that seemed to best capture the constructs of interest.

Adherence to Asian Cultural Values

Asian Values Scale – Revised (AVS-R) [40] contains 25 items and was developed based on the Asian Values Scale (AVS) [41], a reliable and valid measure of adherence to Asian cultural values. Sample items from the AVS-R are "One should not deviate from familial and social norms," and "One should be discouraged from talking about one's accomplishments." The instrument contains 12 negatively worded Asian values statements that are reverse-scored for data analysis. Although it contains fewer items, the AVS-R represents a psychometric improvement over the AVS. To develop the AVS-R, BSK Kim and Hong (2004) [40] used the Rasch model (1960) [42] to first examine the 7-point anchor of the AVS to determine whether it represented the full range of responses well. Three of these categories were found to be an inadequate representation of the responses. For example, the anchor point 4 (*neither agree nor disagree*) may not be conceived as a halfway point between the anchor point 1 and anchor point 7, and may represent item irrelevancy. Consequently, the 7-point anchor was changed to a 4-point scale (1 = strongly disagree, 2 = disagree, 3 = agree, and 4 = strongly agree). Second, the infit and outfit statistics were used to identify and delete 11 items, 7 of which were found to contribute to a decrease in the measure's construct homogeneity and 4 items that were redundant with other items. Despite the removal of nearly one-third of the items, the AVS-R retained the same level of internal consistency as the AVS, with a person separation reliability (a Rasch model analog of Cronbach's α) of 0.80. An examination of the final 25 items that were retained from the AVS indicated that they functioned well to represent the full range of "person trait level" (i.e., the degrees to which the respondents adhered to Asian cultural values) and "item difficulty level" (i.e., likelihood of endorsement for each item). As for the present data, Cronbach's α of 0.72 for children's scores and 0.81 for actual parents' score were observed. For the full AVS scale, please see the appendix.

Cognitive flexibility. The Cognitive Flexibility Scale (CFS) [27] is a 12-item self-report measure of cognitive flexibility. Sample items include "I can communicate an idea in many different ways" and "I can find workable solutions to seemingly unsolvable problems." The CFS is anchored on a 6-point Likert-type scale (1=*strongly disagree* to 6 = *strongly agree*). Four of the scale items are worded negatively and are reverse-scored. Regarding validity, Martin and Rubin (1995) [27] reported significant positive correlation between CFS scores and the scores on a measure of communication flexibility and a significant negative correlation between CFS scores and the scores on a measure of attitude rigidity. Furthermore, using data from another sample, Martin and Rubin reported additional evidence of CFS scores' construct validity in the scale's correlations with scores on measures of interpersonal attentiveness, perceptiveness, and responsiveness, of self-monitoring, and of unwillingness to communicate. Martin and Rubin (1995) [27] reported coefficient α of 0.76 and 0.77 across two samples, suggesting internal consistency of the scale's score. In addition, Martin and Rubin reported a coefficient of stability of 0.83 across a

1-week period, suggesting test–retest reliability of the scale's scores. The present data yielded a coefficient α of 0.76 for children's scores.

Parent–child conflicts. The Intergenerational Conflict Inventory (ICI) [19] is a 24-item measure of intergenerational conflicts in Asian American families. The scale is intended for Asian American young adults to indicate the degree to which they experience a conflict with their parents regarding various types of issues. Across the 24 items, a factor analysis yielded a three-factor solution, leading to the establishment of subscales: expectations about the relationship with family (ICI-Family Expectations; 11 items); education and career (ICI-Education and Career; 10 items); and dating and marriage (ICI-Dating and Marriage; 3 items). Sample items within the area of ICI-Family Expectations are "lack of communication with your parent," "following cultural traditions," and "pressure to learn one's own Asian language." Sample items for ICI-Education and Career are "how much time to spend on studying," "importance of academic achievement," "which career to pursue," and "being compared to others." Sample items for ICI-Dating and Marriage are "Whom to date" and "when to marry." For each item, participants respond on a 6-point Likert-type scale ranging from 1 (*no conflict over this issue*) to 6 (*a lot of conflict over this issue*). Chung (2001) [19] reported adequate internal consistency for the ICI subscale scores: ICI-Family Expectations (coefficient $\alpha=0.86$), ICI-Education and Career (coefficient $\alpha=0.88$), and ICI-Dating and Marriage (coefficient $\alpha=0.84$). In addition, a adequate test–retest reliability across 7 weeks was observed for the subscales with the coefficients of stability ranging from 0.81 to 0.87. Chung (2001) [19] also reported ICI score' evidence of face validity through an examination by high school students and counselor trainees ($N = 10$) who identified the measure as referring to possible sources of tensions between respondents and their parents. Based on the data from the children, the observed Cronbach's α were 0.93 for ICI-Total, 0.84 for ICI-Family Expectations, 0.92 for ICI-Education and Career, and 0.92 for ICI-Dating and Marriage.

Procedure

Because the sample included predominantly first-generation Korean American parents who tend to have limited English language proficiency, the instruments for the parent version were translated utilizing a forward–backward translation method [43]. One translator was involved in the process of first translating the original English version of the instruments into Korean and another translator then translated the Korean version back to English. The original English version and the retranslated English version were compared to examine the accuracy of the Korean translations. For discrepancies between the original version and the translated version, the final translator reconciled them by making changes to the Korean version. All translators were bilingual individuals proficient in both English and Korean.

Prior to data collection, approvals from the institutional review board of the host institution and instructors/leaders of solicited locations were secured.

Solicited locations included Korean-related academic courses (i.e., Korean history, Korean language, and Asian American psychology), Korean-related student organizations (i.e., Korean American Campus Missions, Korean Cultural Awareness Group, and Korean Student Association), Educational Opportunity Program, Resource Center for Sexual and Gender Diversity, and Korean churches. In addition, participants were recruited through flyer advertisements and emails that asked Korean American students to come to a research office at a designated time to complete the questionnaire. A monetary incentive of $5 was offered to these students. No incentive was given to students recruited from some courses and churches. All participants were informed about the anonymous and voluntary nature of participation.

The child participants were given the following instructions before filling out their own questionnaire. They were asked to write their parents' name and addresses on a large stamped envelope that was mailed later to parents. Where the return address was located, the child participants wrote their name for parents to recognize from which child the survey came. There was also a place on the upper left corner for child participants to check whether they thought their parents would prefer an English or Korean version. The researchers also gave the child participants a stamped reminder card. On this card, they were asked to write their names on the back of the reminder card and their parents' names and addresses on the front. After the researchers collected the completed questionnaires from each child participant, the matching parent survey was mailed along with an informed consent and a stamped return envelope. The instructions on the survey asked the parent to complete the survey based on both parents' collective attitudes. A pen with a university logo stamped on it was included in the mailing packet as an incentive for the parents. Two weeks later, a reminder card was mailed to the parents to remind them to turn in their survey.

Results

Preliminary Analysis

The means, standard deviations, and intercorrelations of the study's variables are presented in Table 1.

Remuneration or no remuneration. An examination of the dependent variables for possible relations with whether or not the respondents received a monetary incentive indicated no differences for all variables: ICI-Total [$t(143) = -0.34, P = 0.736$], ICI-Family Expectations [$t(143) = -0.76, P = 0.449$], ICI-Education and Career [$t(143) = -0.17, P = 0.863$], and ICI-Dating and Marriage [$t(143) = 0.36, P = 0.723$]. Hence, data were combined with respect to this variable.

Table 1 Means, standard deviations, and intercorrelations for the predictor and criterion variables

Variable	M	SD	A	B	C	D	E	F	G
A. AVS-R Child	2.49	0.28	–						
B. AVS-R Parent	2.54	0.29	0.06	–					
C. AVS-R Gap	0.04	0.39	–0.68***	0.69***	–				
D. CFS Child	4.44	0.58	–0.13	0.11	0.17*	–			
E. ICI-Total Child	2.77	1.00	0.00	0.10	0.07	–0.16	–		
F. ICI-FE Child	2.53	0.93	–0.20*	0.05	0.18*	–0.04	0.88***	–	
G. ICI-EC Child	3.06	1.34	0.09	0.11	–0.02	–0.25	0.90***	0.63	–
H. ICI-DM Child	2.67	1.64	0.03	0.07	0.03	–0.03	0.60***	0.47***	0.35***

*$P < 0.05$; **$P < 0.01$; and ***$P < 0.001$.

Residence with or without parents. An examination of the dependent variables for possible relations with whether or not the respondents currently lived with their parents indicated no differences for all variables: ICI-Total [$t(142) = 1.00$, $P = 0.322$], ICI-Family Expectations [$t(142) = 0.97$, $P = 0.333$], ICI-Education and Career [$t(142) = 1.09$, $P = 0.278$], and ICI-Dating and Marriage [$t(142) = -0.04$, $P = 0.972$]. Hence, data were combined with respect to this variable.

Age. There were no significant relationships between age and ICI-Total ($r = -0.02$, $P > 0.05$), ICI-Family Expectations ($r = 0.05$, $P > 0.05$), ICI-Education and Career ($r = -0.08$, $P > 0.05$), and ICI-Dating and Marriage ($r = 0.06$, $P > 0.05$). Hence, data were combined with respect to this variable

Gender and generation. To assess for the effects of gender and generation level of the child on the parent–child conflict variables, a multivariate analysis of variance was conducted. Gender and generation were entered as independent variables with ICI scores as dependent variables. There was no main effect for gender, Wilks' $l = 0.989$, $F(4, 135) = 0.37$, $P = 0.828$. There was also no main effect for generation level, Wilks' $l = 0.962$, $F(14, 135) = 1.33$, $P = 0.263$. Hence, data were combined with respect to these variables.

Calculation of the parent–child values gap score. To calculate the parent-child values gap score, each child's AVS-R score was subtracted from the parent's AVS-R scores.

Main Analyses

For the main purpose of the study, the correlational analysis indicated a significant relation between the parent–child values gap score and ICI-Family Expectations ($r = 0.18$, $P < 0.05$). However, no significant relations were found between the values gap score and the other ICI scores.

As for the secondary purpose of the study in examining the possible moderating role of a child's cognitive flexibility, four hierarchical multiple regression analyses were conducted, one for each of the ICI scores (ICI-Total, ICI-Family Expectations, ICI-Education and Career, and ICI-Dating and Marriage). In step 1, the independent variable of child–parent Asian values gap and the moderating variable of cognitive flexibility were entered. In step 2, the interaction term produced by multiplying the child–parent Asian values gap score and the cognitive flexibility score were entered. In creating this interaction term, the variables were centered to reduce the possibility of multicollinearity.

The results indicated a significant overall equation for ICI-Education and Career (see Table 2); the other dependent variables did not yield significant regression equations. The standardized β-coefficient for the interaction variable indicated a significant moderator effect for cognitive flexibility. Interestingly, further examination of the interaction effect showed that for children with high cognitive flexibility, there was a positive relationship between child–parent values gap and child-reported frequency of conflicts in the area of education and career (see Fig. 1). For children with low cognitive flexibility, there was a negative relationship between child–parent values gap and child-reported frequency of education and career conflicts.

Discussion of the Results

The present study yielded a significant positive relationship between the child–parent Asian values gap and child-reported conflict in the area of expectations about family relationships. This result is consistent with existing literature that suggests that the parent–child gap in cultural values is associated with parent–child conflict [19, 20, 29, 39]. For example, Ahn et al. (2005) [29] found that the Korean American child-perceived Asian values gap between themselves and their parents was significantly related to increased frequency of conflicts in the areas of education and career as well as dating and marriage. Although the present findings were not identical to those of Ahn et al. in terms of the area of conflicts, the findings provide support for the theory that increased cultural values gap between parents and children is associated with increased conflicts in

Table 2 Results of hierarchical multiple regression analyses of Asian values gap and child's cognitive flexibility on ICI-education and career

	b	t	P	R^2	F	P	ΔR^2
Step 1				0.06	4.68	0.011	0.06
Values Gap (A)	0.03	0.32	0.748				
Cognitive Flexibility (B)	−0.25	−3.05	0.003				
Step 2				0.09	4.74	0.004	0.03
AVS-R Gap (A)	0.00	−0.05	0.961				
Child's CFS (B)	−0.27	−3.30	0.001				
A X B	0.18	2.15	0.034				

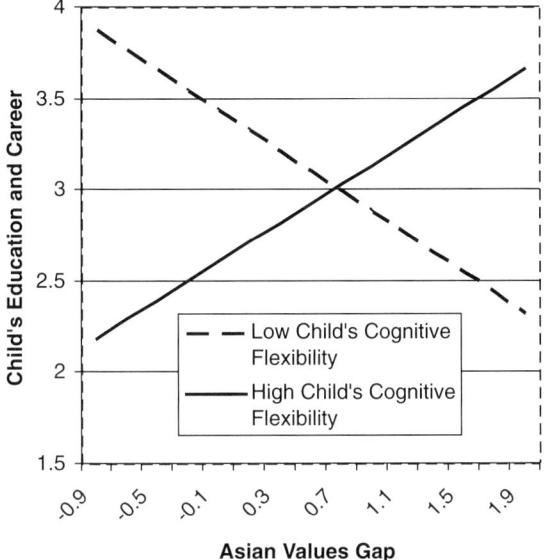

Fig. 1 Interaction effect between Asian values gap and child's cognitive flexibility on child-reported education and career conflict

the family. Furthermore, in terms of the salience of the area of expectations about family relationships among Korean Americans, Chung (2001) [19] found that Korean American college students experienced more conflicts in the area of family expectations in comparison with Japanese American students.

The present study also examined a child's cognitive flexibility as a possible moderator on the relationships between parent–child Asian values gap and parent–child conflicts in the areas of expectations about family relationships, education and career, and dating and marriage. The results showed that cognitive flexibility served as a moderator in the positive relationship between Asian values gap and child-reported education and career conflict. However, contrary to previous literature, the direction of the interaction was reversed: children with high cognitive flexibility tended to have increased conflict as the values gap increased, whereas children with low cognitive flexibility tended to have decreased conflict. Although it is difficult to explain this unexpected finding, one possible explanation lies in the correlational nature of the present study. Perhaps this result indicates that due to increased Asian value differences and the frequency of conflict over education and career choices, children respond with high cognitive flexibility. In other words, children may be using higher levels of cognitive flexibility in an attempt to deal with the intense level of value differences with their parents, which in turn influences the frequency of conflict. When Asian values gap is not considered at various levels, cognitive flexibility was associated with a decreased level of education and career conflicts.

Another possible explanation is that there may be ways in which cognitive flexibility backfires and creates more conflict when there are large Asian value differences. This interpretation can be elaborated with the findings in the study of Martin et al (1998) [44]. These authors found that the use of cognitive flexibility was related to the characteristics of communication competence, which included assertiveness, argumentation, and responsiveness among college students. Initially, this study's result appeared to set a good rationale for cognitive flexibility decreasing the levels of conflict due to the elements of communication competence. However, it could be that those aspects of communication may be effective, but only selectively with Asian American children and parents who are more acculturated (45). To further elaborate, Gudykunst (2001) [46] described the existence of cross-cultural differences in communication styles between Western and Eastern cultures. For Western cultures, the author used the term low-context communication style to describe the specific, precise, and direct modes of communication that are expressed when transmitting messages. These aspects have similar elements of communication competence that was described above. However, this communication style may not be cross-culturally effective in the dynamic between Korean American children and their traditional Korean parents. In fact, it may cause cultural clashes because traditional Asian parents may expect their children to adhere to high-context communication style, which is described as indirect, implicit, and polite approaches to sending messages. The author characterized high-context communication style in relation to traditional Asian collectivistic values and its maintenance of social hierarchy. Therefore, when children use high cognitive flexibility in the face of high Asian values gap and conflict, they could be perceived as expressing their views in a manner that threatens this hierarchy, thereby exacerbating the frequency of conflicts.

Limitations and Implications

The findings in the current study have limitations that are typical of survey research with university students. Although a significant proportion of Korean Americans with whom counselors are likely to work with will be college students, the use of these individuals in the present study limits the generalizability of findings to Korean Americans not in college settings. Similarly, the results may apply only to college students in the West Coast and not the other geographical areas, and not apply to other Asian American ethnic groups. The study was also selective in gathering data from parents who turned in their survey, making it difficult for random sampling. In addition, given that we asked the respondent to represent the views of their spouse, the results might be different if we asked mothers and fathers separately.

Despite these limitations, there are several research implications. As the present study focused only on children's perceptions of parent–child conflict and their cognitive flexibility, future studies should also focus on the perceptions of parents in terms of their conflicts with their children and their cognitive flexibility. In addition, given that the present study examined only the values gap relative to the Asian culture, future studies should also examine values gap regarding adherence to mainstream US culture (i.e., acculturation). An instrument that may be helpful in this regard is the *European American Values Scale for Asian Americans – Revised* [47], a measure of values acculturation. In addition, it is recommended to assess the differences in acculturation and enculturation in other dimensions, such as behaviors, knowledge, and racial ethnic identity. In future studies, it may also be useful to include a measure of social desirability, because family shame may play a role in how much parents and children disclose about the conflicts between them. For the full scale, please see the appendix.

In terms of clinical implications, given some of the significant relations among parent–child Asian values gap, cognitive flexibility, and intergenerational conflicts, clinicians may profit from exploring these variables with their parent–child clients. Doing so could help to illuminate the intrapersonal and interpersonal dynamics that may exist between the clients. As these dynamics are known, clinicians could help clients develop new strategies to successfully cope with their problems and avoid future ones.

Conclusion

In this chapter, we described the construct definitions of acculturation and enculturation and explored the psychological theories and research on these two constructs as related to Asian American families. Then, we described the findings from a recently completed study focusing on values enculturation among Korean Americans, a significant subpopulation among Asian Americans.

Through this chapter, we hope to have created a greater appreciation for the within-group variability among Asian American families in terms of acculturation and enculturation. In addition, we hope that the readers have increased their understanding about the potential pitfalls that exist for Asian American families as they engage in adapting to the norms of the dominant US culture while trying to retain the norms of their Asian ethnic culture. In particular, it is important to be aware of the serious pitfalls in the form of parent–child conflict as a result of the differential adherences to traditional Asian values between parents and children and the moderating role of a child's cognitive flexibility. Through this type of understanding, we hope that the clinicians can increase their effectiveness when working with Asian American families.

References

1. Redfield R, Linton R, Herskovits, MJ. Memorandum on the study of acculturation. American Anthropologist 1936; 56: 973–1002.
2. Graves TD. Psychological acculturation in a tri-ethnic community. Southwestern J Anthropol 1967; 23: 337–350.

3. Berry JW. Acculturation as varieties of adaptation. In: Padilla AM, ed. *Acculturation: Theory, Models, and Some New Findings*. Boulder, CO: Westview Press, 1980: pp. 9–25.
4. Segall MH, Dasen PR, Berry JW, Poortinga YH. *Human Behavior in Global Perspective: An Introduction to Cross-Cultural Psychology*. New York: Pergamon Press, 1999.
5. Herskovits MJ. *Man and his Works: The Science of Cultural Anthropology*. New York: Knopf, 1948.
6. Kim BSK. Acculturation and enculturation. In: Leong FTL, Inman AG, Ebreo A, Yang L, Kinoshita L, Fu M, eds. *Handbook of Asian American Psychology*, 2nd ed. Thousand Oaks, CA: Sage, 2007: pp. 141–158.
7. Kim BSK, Abreu JM. Acculturation measurement: Theory, current instruments, and future directions. In: Ponterotto, JG, Casas JM, Suzuki, LA, Alexander, CM, eds. *Handbook of Multicultural Counseling*, 2nd ed., Thousand Oaks, CA: Sage, 2001: pp. 394–424.
8. Kim, BSK, Atkinson, DR, and Umemoto, D. Asian cultural values and the counseling process: Current knowledge and directions for future research. Couns Psychol 2001; 29:570–603.
9. Szapocznik, J, Scopetta, MA, Kurtines, W, Aranalde, MA. Theory and measurement of acculturation. InterAm J Psychol 1978; 12: 113–120.
10. Sodowsky, GR, Maestas, MV. Acculturation, ethnic identity, and acculturative stress: Evidence and measurement. In: Dana, R ed. *Handbook of Cross-Cultural and Multicultural Personality Assessment*, Mahwah, NJ: Lawrence Erlbaum, 2000: pp. 131–172.
11. Hwang, W. Acculturative family distancing: Theory, research and clinical practice. *Psychotherapy Theory, Research, Practice, Training* 2007; 43: pp. 397–409.
12. Rosenthal, DA, Demtriou, A, Efklides, A. A cross-national study of the influence of culture on conflict between parents and adolescents. Int J Behav Dev 1989; 12: 207–219.
13. Matsuoka, JK. Differential acculturation among Vietnamese refugees. Soc Work 1990; 35: 341–345.
14. Szapocznik, J, Kurtines, WM. Family psychology and cultural diversity: Opportunities for theory, research, and applications. Am Psychol 1993; 48: 400–407.
15. Dasgupta, SD. Gender roles and cultural continuity in the Asian Indian immigrant community in the U.S. Sex Roles 1998; 38: 953–973.
16. Uba, L. *Asian Americans*. New York: Guilford Press, 1994.
17. Portes, A. Immigration theory for a new century: Some problems and opportunities. Int Migr Rev 1997; 31: 799–825.
18. Ryu, JP, Vann, BH. Korean families in America. In: Procidana, ME, Fischer, CB eds. In: *Contemporary Families: A Handbook for School Professionals*, New York, NY: Teachers College Press, 1992: 117–134.
19. Chung, RHG. Gender, ethnicity, and acculturation in intergenerational conflict of Asian American college students. Cultur Divers Ethnic Minor Psychol 2001; 7: 376–386.
20. Lee, JC, Cynn, VEH. Issues in 1.5 generation Korean Americans. In: Lee, C, Richardson, B eds. *Multicultural Issues in Counseling: New Approaches to Diversity*, Alexandria, VA: American Association for Counseling and Development, 1991: 127–140.
21. Lee, RM, Choe, J, Kim, G, Ngo, V. Construction of the Asian American Family Conflict Scale. J Couns Psychol 2000; 47: 211–222.
22. Phinney, JS, Ong, A, Madden, T. Cultural values and intergenerational value discrepancies in immigrant and non-immigrant families. Child Dev 2000; 71: 528–539.
23. Kim, JM. Structural family therapy and its implications for the Asian American families. Fam J2003; 11(4): 388–392.
24. LaFromboise, T, Coleman, H, Gerton, J. Psychological impact of biculturalism: Evidence and theory. Psychol Bull 1993; 114: 395–412.
25. Berry, JW, Annis, RC. Acculturative stress: The role of ecology, culture, and differentiation. J Cross Cult Psychol 1974; 5: 382–406.

26. Nguyen, HH, Messe, LA, Stollak, GE. Toward a more complex understanding of acculturation and adjustment: Cultural involvements and psychosocial functioning in Vietnamese youth. J Cross Cult Psychol 1999; 30(1): 5–31.
27. Martin, MM, Rubin, RB. A new measure of cognitive flexibility. Psychol Rep 1995; 76, 623–626.
28. Harrison, AO, Wilson, MN, Pine, CJ, Chan, SQ. Family ecologies of ethnic minority children. Child Dev 1990; 60: 347–362.
29. Ahn, AJ, Kim BSK, Park YS. Asian cultural values gap and child–parent conflict among Korean Americans. Poster session presented at the annual meeting of the American Psychological Association, Washington, D.C.:2005.
30. Atkinson, DR. ed. *Counseling American Minorities*, 6th ed., Boston: McGraw-Hill, 2004.
31. Sue, DW, Sue, D. ed. *Counseling the Culturally Different: Theory and Practice*, 4th ed., New York, NY: John Wiley & Sons, 2003.
32. Chan, KS, Hune, S. Racialization and panethnicity: From Asians in America to Asian Americans. In: Hawley, WD, Anthony, JW. Eds. *Toward a Common Destiny: Improving Race Relationships in America*, San Francisco, CA: Jossey-Bass Inc., 1995: 205–233.
33. Wakil, SP, Siddique, CM, Wakil, FA. Between two cultures: A study in socialization of children of immigrants. J Marriage Fam 1981; 43: 929–940.
34. Nguyen, NA, Williams, HL. Transition from East to West: Vietnamese adolescents and their parents. J Am Acad Child Child Adolesc Psychiatry 1989; 28: 505–515.
35. Rosenthal, DA. Intergenerational conflict and culture: A study of immigrant and non-immigrant adolescents and their parents. Genet Psychol Monogr 1984; 109: 53–75.
36. Rosenthal, D, Ranieri, N, Kimidis, S. Vietnamese adolescents in Australia: Relationships between perceptions of self and parental values, intergenerational conflict, and gender dissatisfaction. Int J Psychol 1996; 31(2): 81–91.
37. Kwak, K, Berry, J. Generational differences in acculturation among Asian families in Canada: A comparison of Vietnamese, Korean and East-Indian groups. Int J Psych 2001; 36:152–162.
38. Lowinger, RJ, Kwok, H. Parental overprotection in Asian American children: A psychodynamic clinical perspective. Psychotherapy 2001; 38: 319–330.
39. Rohner, RP, Pettengill, SM. Perceived parental acceptance-rejection and parental control among Korean adolescents. Child Dev 1985; 56: 524–528.
40. Kim, BSK, Hong, S. A psychometric revision of the Asian Values Scale using the Rasch model. Meas Eval Couns Dev 2004; 37:15–27.
41. Kim, BSK, Atkinson, D, Yang, PH. The Asian Value Scale: Development, Factor Analysis, Validation, and Reliability. J Couns Psychol 1999; 46: 342–352.
42. Rasch, G. *Probabilistic Models for Some Intelligence and Attainment Tests*. Chicago: Mesa Press, 1960.
43. Brislin, R. Back translation for cross-cultural research. J Cross Cult Psych 1970; 1: 185
44. Martin, MM, Anderson, CM, Thweatt, KS. Aggressive communication traits and their relationships with the cognitive flexibility scale and the communication flexibility scale. J Soc Behav Pers 1998; 13(3): 531–540.
45. Kim, BSK, Omizo, MM. Asian and European American cultural values, collective self-esteem, acculturative stress, cognitive flexibility, and general self-efficacy among Asian American college students. J Couns Psychol 2005; 52(3): 412–419.
46. Gudykunst, WB. *Asian American Ethnicity and Communication*. Thousand Oaks, CA: Sage Publications, Inc., 2001.
47. Hong, S, Kim, BSK, Wolfe, MM. A psychometric revision of the European American Values Scale for Asian Americans using the Rasch model. Meas Eval Couns Dev 2005; 37: 194–207.

Strengthening Intergenerational/Intercultural Ties in Immigrant Families (SITIF): A Parenting Intervention to Bridge the Chinese American Intergenerational Acculturation Gap

Yu-Wen Ying

Abstract Intergenerational and intercultural conflict is a significant stressor in immigrant families that occurs because of differential acculturation between migrant parents and their children. In spite of its negative mental health consequences, few empirically tested interventions address this problem. Strengthening Intergenerational/Intercultural Ties in Immigrant Families (SITIF) is a culturally sensitive, community-based intervention that aims to strengthen the intergenerational relationship. It promotes immigrant parents' emotional awareness and empathy for their children's experiences, cognitive knowledge and understanding of differences between their native and American cultures, and teaches behavioral parenting skills with the objective of enhancing intergenerational intimacy. SITIF was tested with a group of 16 middle class and 14 working class immigrant Chinese parents. Using objective and subjective assessment tools, the findings provide empirical support for SITIF's effectiveness in enhancing parenting skills and strengthening the intergenerational relationship in immigrant Chinese American families.

Keywords SITIF · Intergenerational/intercultural conflict · Immigrant families · Culturally sensitive community-based intervention · Chinese American immigrants · Asian American families

Contents
Strengthening Intergenerational/Intercultural Ties in Immigrant Families 46
Significance of Intergenerational/Intercultural Conflict in Immigrant Families 47
Strengthening Intergenerational/Intercultural Ties in Immigrant Families (SITIF) . . . 48

This chapter is adapted from Ying, Y. Strengthening Intergenerational/Intercultural Ties in Immigrant Families (SITIF): A culturally-sensitive community-based intervention with Chinese American parents. J Immigr Refug Stud 2007; 5: 67–90.

Y.-W. Ying (✉)
School for Social Welfare, 120 Haviland Hall, University of California, Berkeley, CA 94720-7400, USA
e-mail: ywying10@berkeley.edu

SITIF's Effectiveness with Chinese American Immigrant Parents 50
Method 52
  Sample 52
  Procedure 53
  Measures 54
Results 56
  Engagement with SITIF 56
  Objective Mastery of the SITIF Curriculum 56
  Subjective Evaluation of SITIF's Effectiveness 57
  Association of and Objective Mastery and Subjective Evaluation
    of Effectiveness 59
Discussion 59
  Engagement with SITIF 59
  Objective Mastery of the SITIF Curriculum 60
  Subjective Evaluation of SITIF's Effectiveness 61
  Association of Objective Mastery and Subjective Evaluation of Effectiveness 61
  Study Limitations and Directions for Future Research 61
References 62

Strengthening Intergenerational/Intercultural Ties in Immigrant Families

Testing a culturally sensitive, community-based intervention with Chinese American parents

A quarter of a century ago, Sluzki [1] identified intergenerational conflict as a significant problem in immigrant families. Owing to developmental variation in susceptibility to environmental influences and differential opportunities to engage with American culture through schooling and peers, immigrant and American-born children of immigrants acculturate more quickly to the United States than their parents who migrated as adults [1–10]. This gap in acculturation has been identified as a key contributor to intergenerational conflict in immigrant families [6, 9, 11–13]. Thus, Ho [14] found that, in spite of Chinese culture's greater emphasis on intergenerational harmony, first- and second-generation Chinese American adolescents with immigrant parents report more intergenerational conflict than their European American peers from non-immigrant families [15]. Among children of immigrants, intergenerational conflict is particularly prominent among adolescents who are engaged in the developmental task of separation and individuation from their parents [3–5, 8, 9, 16]. In particular, conflict is greater among those who migrated by the age of 12 years or were born in the United States compared with those who migrated after age 12 years and were less acculturated to US mainstream culture [17], those from working than from middle class families [6], and among girls than among boys [18, 19]. It is also possible that the degree of intergenerational conflict differs by the pathway of adaptation employed by children of immigrants who assimilate to varying segments of American society – for example, white middle class, the inner-city underclass, or solidarity within their ethnic community [20–22].

In spite of the significant research that documents intergenerational conflict in immigrant families, very few interventions are available to ameliorate this problem. A notable exception is the series of interventions developed by Szapocznik and his colleagues [23], which will be discussed below. The current study contributes to the intervention literature for immigrant families by testing a culturally sensitive, community-based intervention, Strengthening Intergenerational/Intercultural Ties in Immigrant Families (SITIF), with Chinese American parents. The significance of intergenerational/intercultural conflict in immigrant families is presented below, followed by a description of SITIF, and an empirical study that assesses its utility in middle and working class Chinese American immigrants.

Significance of Intergenerational/Intercultural Conflict in Immigrant Families

Intergenerational/intercultural conflict in immigrant families is a significant problem for a number of reasons. First, because of the sheer size of the immigrant population, the number of individuals potentially affected by this problem is considerable. At the dawn of the twenty-first century, immigrants comprise 12% of the American population and number 32.5 million [24]. In the state of California, where SITIF was developed, immigrants already comprise over a quarter of the population [25]. Unlike a century ago, the majority of today's immigrants originate not from Europe but from Asia and Latin America [24]. Consequently, over half of Latino and 88% of Asian children nationwide are growing up in immigrant households [22]. Therefore, 20% of American youth have at least one parent who is non-native born [26] and are at risk of experiencing intergenerational/intercultural conflict.

Second, although the prevalence of intergenerational/intercultural conflict in immigrant families is unknown, it is likely to be a common problem. Asian and Latin American cultural values vary significantly from those of the majority culture; American schools and mass media espouse majority culture values, and thus promote them to the children of immigrants. For instance, whereas independence and individual uniqueness are valued in mainstream American culture, Asian and Latin American cultures emphasize interdependence and interpersonal harmony [14, 27]. Within the intergenerational relationship, Latin American and Asian parents are generally more authoritarian than their European American counterparts. In addition, the parent–child bond is more hierarchical and lifelong in Latin American and Asian cultures, whereas it is more egalitarian in European American families where children are expected to separate and individuate during adolescence [2, 28, 29]. Such divergent values are likely to lead to significant intergenerational incongruence when children progressively acculturate to the host country's values, attitudes, and behaviors, while parents continue to embrace their home culture. As noted above, empirical research shows that less-acculturated immigrant parents [11, 13] and more-acculturated children of immigrants [6, 9, 16, 17] report more intergenerational incongruence. Even when children of immigrants do espouse their ethnic culture, they may be viewed as "not ethnic enough" according to parental standards [29].

Third, intergenerational/intercultural conflict in immigrant families is significant because of the psychological distress it inflicts on both immigrant parents and their children [5]. A major motivator for migration is the hope for a better life for the next generation. Although many of the migration-related challenges, such as culture shock, economic difficulties, and discrimination, may be anticipated, immigrants rarely expect nor prepare for intergenerational/intercultural discord [30, 31]. When it occurs, parents feel dismayed and betrayed [8, 28]. For immigrant parents from Latin American and Asian cultures where intimate intergenerational ties is the norm and highly valued, such conflict may be especially painful [32]. Concurrently, the child of immigrants may feel confused and trapped by the conflicting home and school/societal cultures, and the inconsistent values and expectations of parents and peers, resulting in depression, anxiety, gang involvement, and academic difficulties and failure [9, 19, 23, 33–35].

Strengthening Intergenerational/Intercultural Ties in Immigrant Families (SITIF)

SITIF is a community-based educational intervention that aims to strengthen the intergenerational relationship between immigrant parents and their school age children and adolescents. SITIF may be used as a primary or secondary prevention as well as tertiary prevention or treatment for intergenerational/intercultural conflict in immigrant families. Informed by Bandura's social learning theory [36], SITIF concurrently targets parents' affect, cognition, and behavior, which may reciprocally influence one another [37]. Specifically, through the intervention, parents learn to affectively empathize with their child's perspective, to cognitively understand variation in the ethnic and American cultures and its impact on their child's development, to recognize a difference in values and their intergenerational relationships, and to develop effective behavioral parenting skills, all of which promote intergenerational communication and intimacy as well as reduce conflict. In addition, parents are introduced to methods adapted from a course on depression prevention [37] that may be used to cope with the stresses of parenting and migration. A detailed instructor's manual and parenting handouts for SITIF curriculum ensure the fidelity of delivery across instructors.

A notable characteristic of SITIF is the incorporation of cultural competency principles in its development, including awareness of cultural differences, knowledge of cultural content (such as norms, customs, language, life style, etc.), accurate assessment and differentiation between culture and pathology (i.e., the culture-bound nature of normality and abnormality), and use of culturally competent interventions [38, 39]. Sue and Zane [40] further specified that the culturally competent clinician achieves credibility and effectiveness by sharing the client's problem conceptualization, means of solution, goal setting, and gift giving; these were also incorporated into the design of SITIF.

SITIF comprises four main parts: [1] increasing awareness of cultural differences between the two generations; [2] increasing knowledge of differences; [3] providing assessments of the difference; and [4] providing an intervention directed at minimizing the differences. SITIF is grounded in the reality that parenting practices vary across cultures (*awareness of cultural difference*), and intergenerational conflict in immigrant families occurs partially due to immigrants' use of parenting methods that are not supported or sanctioned by American culture. For instance, Latin American and Asian immigrant parents may prefer commands and directives, while their children prefer discussion (*knowledge of cultural difference*). Furthermore, SITIF *assesses* intergenerational conflict and attributes it to intercultural difference, not individual pathology, thereby removing blame from both the parent and the child. Finally, SITIF is a culturally sensitive *intervention* that employs a familiar, educational format. It is not presented as a traditional mental health service that ethnic immigrant Americans have been found to underuse due to unfamiliarity, misconceptions, and stigma [41, 42].

In the SITIF curriculum, the parents' awareness of cultural difference is enhanced affectively through a simulated exercise of cross-cultural encounter, and listening to an adult child of immigrants from their ethnic group share her perspective of the intergenerational relationship while growing up. Discussions about the immigrant and majority American cultures' values and norms in general, and specifically with regard to the parent–child relationship, contribute to the parents' growing knowledge of cultural differences. Building on theoretical discussions of acculturation, ethnic identity, and child development, parents learn to assess and understand their child's behavior and the intergenerational relationship in the sociocultural contexts of the ethnic and majority American cultures. Finally, SITIF encourages immigrants to consider culture in their parenting by teaching behavioral parenting skills; these skills help incorporate the child's perspective in problem conceptualization, means of solution, goal setting, and gift giving [40]. All of these components contribute to strengthen the intergenerational relationship.

The parenting skills covered in SITIF were adapted from Bernard and Louise Gurney's work on filial therapy [43, 44] which is grounded in Rogerian client-centered therapy and teaches parents to serve as therapists to their children in order to improve the latter's well-being and enhance intergenerational communication and understanding. This type of therapy is consistent with SITIF's aim to reduce intergenerational and intercultural conflict and to enhance communication, understanding, and intimacy. The parenting skills covered in SITIF are additionally grounded in mainstream American cultural values, to which children of immigrants are exposed and acculturate through formal education, peer relations, and mass media. Immigrant parents are not encouraged to discard ethnically specific parenting methods but to expand their repertoire of skills. Different skills have different objectives. At any given moment, parents are invited to employ the skill that is most likely to yield the desired outcome. For example, although immigrant parents may prefer a hierarchical, unidirectional method of communication that is sanctioned by their ethnic culture, their children may prefer a more interactive style that involves less lecturing and more active listening. The latter method is more likely to elicit communication, mutual understanding, and ultimately a more intimate relationship. All of the methods covered in SITIF focus on parenting process (how to), not specific parenting content (what to). For instance, parents may use a skill to facilitate discussion on dating, but they are not advised on the age at which their child should be allowed to date or whether arranged marriage is desirable.

Although SITIF shares a focus on cognitive understanding of cultural differences, intergenerational communication and parenting skills with the Strengthening Families interventions developed by Jose Szapocznik and colleagues [23] for Cuban and other Latino families, it is intended as a generic intervention to be used with immigrant parents from any country of origin. Although this claim remains to be empirically demonstrated, the curriculum does not make reference to any particular immigrant group. It is deliberately flexible for use with any ethnic group. For example, ethnic fairy tales are employed to illustrate ethnic norms and values in contrast with American cultural values. Although the choice of fairy tale varies by immigrant groups, they adhere to the same principle in that they exemplify cultural teaching and values remains the same [45]. In contrast, Strengthening Families is intended specifically for use with Latino families, and therefore places heavy emphasis on the prevention and management of risk problems more commonly found among Latino adolescents, such as academic failure, substance abuse, gang involvement, and teenage pregnancy. Thus, it is unclear whether these interventions are appropriate for immigrant groups where children may not evidence externalizing problem behaviors as frequently.

SITIF's Effectiveness with Chinese American Immigrant Parents

The current study assesses the use of SITIF with middle and working class Chinese American immigrant parents. Chinese Americans number 2.7 million and comprise the largest Asian ethnic group in the United States [46]. Furthermore, two-thirds of Chinese Americans are immigrants [46]. Previous research assessed SITIF's effectiveness in middle class Chinese American immigrant parents using standardized, quantitative measures and found it to enhance parenting efficacy and responsibility, sense of coherence, and overall quality of the intergenerational relationship [30, 31]. However, the Chinese population in the United States is quite diverse. Although the median family income is $60,000, 13.5% of Chinese Americans live below the poverty line [46]. In light of this heterogeneity, it is important to test SITIF's effectiveness across a diverse range of parents. In response to working class parents' difficulty in completing standardized, quantitative baseline measures that were verbally administered to them in Chinese, a problem that has been documented in previous research with unacculturated Asian Americans [47], the current study utilizes non-standardized, open-ended measures to assess SITIF's effectiveness.

Four major research questions were posed as follows: first, do parents engage in SITIF; second, can parents demonstrate objective mastery over the SITIF curriculum and does this vary by the level of engagement; third, does SITIF enhance effective parenting practices and strengthen the intergenerational relationship based on subjective report; and fourth, is objective mastery positively associated with subjective evaluation of the course? Furthermore, across all questions, variation by socioeconomic status is assessed.

With regard to the first research question, to benefit from SITIF, parents must first engage and participate in the intervention. As the literature has repeatedly documented location and hours of operation as potential barriers to ethnic minorities' use of social services [41, 42], SITIF is offered at familiar and centrally located community agencies (e.g., that are situated in Chinatown) and at times convenient for the parents (e.g., concurrent with their children attending Chinese language school). Engagement with the intervention is operationalized primarily by attendance and secondarily by homework completion. The second question examines the retention of SITIF's content, a method commonly used in educational settings to assess mastery of the curriculum. Specifically, parents are asked to respond to questions regarding concepts/techniques covered in class. It is expected that greater engagement would be associated with greater retention of content. The third question assesses the intervention's utility through participants' subjective report of desired behavioral change [48]. Specifically, they are asked to provide an overall assessment of SITIF, and to report postintervention changes in parenting method and the intergenerational relationship. Finally, it is expected that objective mastery of the curriculum would be associated with subjective reports of satisfaction. All four questions are assessed for the entire sample and separately for middle class and working class parents. It is expected that, compared with working class parents, middle class parents are more likely to have better English skills and enjoy more exposure to majority American society, and therefore possess more awareness and knowledge of cultural differences prior to participating in the intervention. Thus, documenting potential variation by socioeconomic status holds implications for whether SITIF may be successfully taught to and utilized by both middle class and working class parents.

Method

Sample

A total of 30 Chinese American parents participated in the study: 16 middle class, Mandarin-speaking parents and 14 working class, Cantonese-speaking parents. Inclusion in the two socioeconomic groups was defined by education and occupation. Table 1 shows the demographic background of the whole sample and the two groups. χ^2 Tests were used to assess variation on categorical variables, and independent t-tests were used to assess difference on continuous variables. The more conservative two-tailed test was used in all analyses. As anticipated, middle class parents were significantly better educated than working class parents (mean = 17.94 years, $SD = 2.41$ vs. mean = 10.86 years, $SD = 3.51$, $t = 6.36$, df = 22.61, $P = 0.001$). They also held higher status jobs than working class parents, as 62.5% of the former were professionals compared with none of the latter. In addition, almost two-thirds of the working class parents (64.3%) were homemakers as compared with 6.3% of the middle class parents ($\chi^2 = 18.01$, df = 3, $P = 0.001$).

Table 1 Demographic characteristics

		All ($n=30$)	Middle class ($n=16$)	working class ($n=14$)
Mean education (SD)***		14.63 (4.63)	17.94 (2.41)	10.86 (3.51)
Occupation***	Professional (%)	33.3	62.5	0
	Business (%)	20	25	14.3
	Clerical (%)	13.3	6.3	21.4
	Homemaker (%)	33.3	6.3	64.3
Sex	Female (%)	83.3	81.3	85.7
Mean age (SD)		41.97 (7.08)	42 (5.93)	41.93 (8.43)
Birth place***	Taiwan (%)	36.7	68.8	0
	China (%)	33.3	12.5	57.1
	Hong Kong (%)	16.7	12.5	21.4
	Other (%)	13.3	6.3	21.4
Mean age at migration (years) (SD)**		28.23 (7.64)	24.63 (3.14)	32.36 (9.20)
Ethnicity composition	Chinese immigrants (%)	70	81.3	57.1
Social network	Mixed (%)	30	18.8	42.9
Mean number of children (SD)		1.90 (0.62)	1.88 (0.72)	1.92 (0.49)
Target child's sex	Male (%)	40	31.3	50
Target child's mean age (years) (SD)		12.50 (6.51)	11 (4.21)	14.21 (8.26)

Significant group differences at *$P<0.05$, **$P<0.01$, ***$P<0.001$, and two-tailed tests.

The two groups also varied on birth place and age at migration. Middle class parents were more likely to be born in Taiwan (68.8%) and working class parents were more likely to be born in China (57.1%; $\chi^2 = 15.74$, df = 3, $P = 0.001$). Middle class parents arrived in the United States at a younger age, most often as graduate students than working class parents who migrated at different ages with a wider distribution (mean = 24.63 years, $SD = 3.14$, range of 20–30 vs. mean = 32.36 years, $SD = 9.20$, range of 22–48, $t = 3.00$, df = 15.64, $P = 0.009$). It can be noted that the mean age of arrival among working class parents was significantly affected by two parents who migrated in their 40s. When the median age of migration for the two groups is compared (i.e., 24 years for middle class parents and 27 years for working class parents), the difference is only 3 years.

The two groups did not vary on sex, age, ethnic composition of social network, and mean number of children. Parents with more than one child were asked to use their oldest child as the target child for homework assignments and assessment questionnaires. The two groups did not vary on the target child's sex and age. Of the participants, 83.3% were female, with a mean age of 41.97 years ($SD = 7.08$). Most reported their social network to be comprised of other Chinese immigrants (70%), whereas the rest had a mix of American-born and overseas-born Chinese friends and/or other Asian friends. On average, the parents had 1.9 children ($SD = 0.62$), with their oldest (or target) child being 12.5 years old (SD = 6.51), and of these 40% were male.

Procedure

Consistent with the dialect preference among Chinese Americans, the middle class parents received the intervention in Mandarin Chinese, whereas the working class parents received the intervention in Cantonese Chinese. The 16 middle class parents were recruited at a presentation on intergenerational conflict held at a Mandarin Chinese language school, whereas the 14 working class parents were recruited by flyers in Chinatown, radio announcements on a Cantonese Chinese community radio talk show, and word of mouth. Upon giving written consent for participation in the evaluation study, parents completed the demographics questionnaire. They then attended the SITIF course. At the last session, parents completed a course evaluation, upon which this report is based.

All classes were held in communities with a high Chinese concentration (areas known as Chinatown), but in two different Northern California cities. The Mandarin-speaking classes were held at a Mandarin Chinese language school on Saturday mornings, whereas the participants' children attended Chinese classes. These classes were closed to newcomers once they began. Mandarin-speaking parents paid $80 in tuition for the SITIF class. The Cantonese-speaking classes were held at a social service agency on a weekday morning, and were offered free of charge. Eight parents who missed the first meeting but dropped in intermittently were accommodated due to the sponsoring agency's policy. On average, they attended 2.88 classes ($SD = 1.36$) but neither signed consent forms nor participated in the evaluation study.

A total of four classes were offered: two for middle class parents and two for working class parents. Each class consisted of meetings lasting 2 h per week over 8 weeks. Detailed class outlines for each class were distributed, and parents were given weekly homework assignments to assist mastery of class content. The course and all measures were administered entirely in Chinese (regardless of spoken dialect, written Chinese remains essentially the same). Consistent with the participants' native and preferred language, middle class parents were taught in Mandarin by the investigator, a native Mandarin-speaking, doctoral-level clinical psychologist, and working class parents were taught in Cantonese by two native Cantonese-speaking, bachelor-level mental health workers who were trained by the investigator and had significant experience serving this population. The use of mental health workers as instructors ensured broad applicability of the intervention [49]. As all instructors followed the same detailed instructor outlines, all parents received the same intervention.

Measures

Two written measures were administered: The Demographics Questionnaire and the SITIF Evaluation Form. The Demographic Questionnaire assessed background information, including education, occupation, sex, age, birthplace, mean at age at migration, ethnic composition of social network, number of children, and target child's sex and age. Parents with more than one child were asked to use their oldest child as the target child, on whom to practice parenting skills as part of their homework assignments. Engagement with SITIF was measured primarily by attendance and secondarily by the completion of homework each week, as recorded by the instructor. Seven sets of homework were assigned over the course of the 8-week intervention. The evaluation measure was developed to assess objective mastery of the curriculum and subjective assessment of its effectiveness.

Objective Mastery over the SITIF Curriculum was assessed on the SITIF Evaluation Form by four domains: awareness/knowledge of cultural differences, rationale/objective of behavioral skills, implementation of skills, and coping with stress. *Awareness/Knowledge* was assessed by a set of five questions: [1] Why does intergenerational/intercultural gap occur in immigrant families? [2] How may immigrant parents learn about differences between Chinese and American cultures? [3] How may immigrant parents participate in the various contexts of their child's life? [4] How may parents assist their children who grow up in the United States with a positive Chinese American identity? [5] How may immigrants serve as culturally competent Chinese American models to their children? Various possible responses to each item were coded as either correct ("1") or incorrect ("0"), yielding a range of possible scores from 0 to 5 for the five items. For instance, a correct response to the first question would cite differential acculturation between the generations. *Rationale/Objective of Behavioral Parenting Skills* was assessed by a set of seven questions that inquired about the aim of skills covered in SITIF: showing understanding, parent's message, structure, reward, rules and limits, punishment, and special time. A sample item was as follows: "What is the rationale/objective of showing understanding? " As above, responses to each item were coded as correct ("1") or incorrect ("0"), which were added up to yield sum scores ranging from 0 to 7. *Implementation of Behavioral Parenting Skills* assessed the procedure of implementing the above seven skills. A sample item was as follows: "How do you show understanding to your child? " The implementation of these skills often involved several steps. As all parents could refer to handouts for details, they were not expected to memorize all the steps. Instead, responses that correctly identified one key step were coded "1." The others were coded "0." Summing their responses to seven items, the range of possible scores was from 0 to 7. Finally, *Coping with Stress* was assessed by the question: How may parents reduce their stress level? Although three methods were covered in SITIF, that is deep breathing, pleasant activities, and social activities, parents were encouraged to choose one or more methods they most enjoyed. Thus, parents who provided at least one of the three methods were coded as "1," and the remainder was coded "0."

Subjective Evaluation of SITIF's Effectiveness was assessed by both closed- and open-ended questions on the SITIF Evaluation Form. The effectiveness score was derived from the responses to seven statements: [1] This course increased my understanding of differences in Chinese and American cultures. [2] This course increased my ability to be a competent Chinese American. [3] This course increased my understanding of my child. [4] This course increased my ability to parent my child. [5] This course increased my communication with my child. [6] This course increased my participation in the various contexts of my child's life. [7] This course increased my connection with my child. They were rated on a 5-point Likert-type scale, with "1" indicating complete disagreement, "3" indicating neutrality, and "5" indicating complete agreement. The overall effectiveness rating was derived from the mean of the seven items. α-Internal reliability of the parenting competence scale was 0.86 for the whole sample, 0.87 for the middle class sample, and 0.84 for the working class sample. Furthermore, parents responded to five open-ended questions that assessed SITIF's effectiveness: As a result of taking this course, [1] How did you change personally? [2] How did you change in the way you parent? [3] What was the most helpful topic we covered? [4] What was the least helpful topic we covered? [5] How did your relationship with your child change?

Based on the curriculum, the researcher developed a code book for the open-ended questions. Two masters level social work students were trained in its use, and independently coded the open-ended responses. One of the coders was a native Mandarin speaker and the other was a native Cantonese speaker who was also fluent in Mandarin. Overall, interrater reliability was 91.8%. Differences were reconciled through discussion.

Results

Engagement with SITIF

Parents' engagement with SITIF was assessed primarily by attendance and secondarily by homework completion. Unless otherwise indicated, independent t-tests were used to assess variation between working and middle class parents across all questions. Two-tailed tests were used. Attendance was very high; of the eight class meetings, the middle class, Mandarin-speaking parents attended an average of 7.5 sessions ($SD = 0.82$) and the working class, Cantonese-speaking parents attended an average of 6.36 ($SD = 1.08$) sessions. Although working class parents attended significantly fewer classes ($t = 3.29$, df = 28, $P = 0.003$), on average, they still attended 80% of the intervention. Thus, both groups of parents engaged significantly with the intervention.

With regard to homework completion, middle class parents completed, on average, 6.19 ($SD = 1.22$) out of 7 sets of homework, again evidencing significant engagement. They wrote their homework and submitted each completed assignment to the instructor for feedback. In contrast, due to lower educational level, working class parents expressed difficulty with writing their homework. Instead, they were encouraged to implement the lessons and report their experience in class verbally. On average, they partially completed about half of the assignments, that is, 3.36 ($SD = 2.84$) sets. The two groups varied significantly in homework completion ($t = 3.45$, df = 17.16, $P = 0.003$).

Objective Mastery of the SITIF Curriculum

To determine objective mastery of the SITIF curriculum, the previously mentioned four domains were assessed: awareness/knowledge, rationale/objective of behavioral parenting skills, implementation of skills, and coping with stress. On average, parents provided 80% correct responses to the awareness/knowledge questions. On the five questions, middle class parents gave, on average, 4.44 ($SD = 0.51$, or 88.8%) correct responses and working class parents gave, on average, 3.79 ($SD = 1.05$ or 75.8%) correct responses (see Table 2). The former significantly outperformed the latter ($t = 2.11$, df = 12.28, $P = 0.05$). Pearson's correlation tests were used to assess association between number of responses given and attendance/homework completion. Greater mastery was associated with attendance ($r = 0.55$, $P = 0.002$) and homework completion ($r = 0.48$, $P = 0.007$). Significant differences on individual items were not found.

Mastery of *Rationale/Objective of Behavioral Parenting Skills* was assessed using seven items, and parents gave an average of 63.33% correct answers. Middle class parents provided 5.06 ($SD = 1.29$ or 72.29%) correct responses, whereas working class parents provided 3.57 ($SD = 1.45$ or 51%) correct responses (see Table 2]. Again, middle class parents demonstrated significantly greater mastery ($t = 2.98$, df=28, $P=0.006$). Attendance also improved mastery

Table 2 Indicators of SITIF's effectiveness

	All (n = 30)	Middle class (n = 16)	Working class (n = 14)
Objective mastery of SITIF (Correct responses (%))			
Mean (SD) Awareness/knowledge (five items)*	4.13 (0.86)	4.44 (0.51)	3.79 (1.05)
Mean (SD) Rationale of skills (seven items)**	4.37 (1.54)	5.06 (1.29)	3.57 (1.45)
Mean (SD) Implementation of skills (seven items)	4.10 (1.77)	4.50 (1.37)	3.64 (2.10)
Mean (SD) Coping with stress (1 item)	0.93 (0.17)	1.00 (0)	0.86 (0.36)
Subjective evaluation of SITIF's effectiveness			
Mean (SD) Effectiveness (seven items)	4.73 (0.34)	4.69 (0.39)	4.78 (0.28)
Reporting personal change (%)	93.3	100	85.7
Reporting parenting method change (%)	90	93.7	85.7
Reporting most helpful topic (%)	90	100	78.6
Reporting least helpful topic (%)	26.7	25	28.5
Reporting improved relationship (%)	96.7	100	92.9

Significant group differences at *$P<0.05$, **$P<0.01$, two-tailed tests.

($r=0.43$, $P=0.02$). Turning to specific items, middle class parents were more likely than working class parents to correctly explain the rationale for showing understanding (87.5 vs. 28.6%, using Fisher's exact test, $P=0.002$) and establishing structure (62.5 vs. 14.3%, using Fisher's exact test, $P=0.011$).

Mastery of *Implementation of Behavioral Parenting Skills* was assessed using seven items. As Table 2 shows, on average, middle class parents provided 4.50 ($SD=1.37$, or 64.28%) correct responses, whereas working class parents provided 3.64 ($SD=2.10$ or 52%) correct responses. Altogether, they gave 56.67% correct answers and did not vary significantly from each other. The number of correct responses increased with attendance ($r=0.39$, $P=0.03$) and homework completion ($r=0.38$, $P=0.04$). In terms of variation on specific items, more middle class parents correctly identified a step in structuring compared with working class parents (75 vs. 28.6%, using Fisher's exact test, $P=0.03$)

Coping with Stress was assessed by one item, and 93.33% gave a correct answer. All of the middle class parents provided at least one correct method, and working class parents provided, on average, 0.86 ($SD=0.36$) correct responses (see Table 2]. Although the two groups did not vary significantly, attendance ($r=0.36$, $P=0.05$) and homework completion ($r=0.41$, $P=0.02$) significantly enhanced mastery.

Subjective Evaluation of SITIF's Effectiveness

Both middle class and working class parents rated the SITIF as extremely effective in enhancing their parenting and strengthening their intergenerational relationship. Using a scale of 1–5, the mean effectiveness rating across the seven closed-ended items was 4.69 ($SD=0.39$) for middle class parents and 4.78 ($SD=0.28$) for working class parents (see Table 2]. The ratings did not vary by either socioeconomic status/language group or engagement (attendance and homework completion). Clearly, the parents found SITIF to be highly effective in enhancing their parenting ability and intergenerational relationship.

Subjective evaluation of effectiveness was also assessed by seven open-ended items, to which multiple, acceptable answers could be given. With regard to *personal change*, 93.3% reported at least one such change consequent to the course (see Table 2]: 40% of the parents were more attentive and willing to consider perspectives other than their own, 70% became better communicators, 13.3% were more aware of Chinese and American cultural differences and/or more accepting of American culture. On average, parents gave a total of 1.57 ($SD=0.77$) responses, and middle and working class parents differed neither on content nor on quantity of responses. Number of responses given also did not vary by engagement with SITIF.

With regard to *parenting method*, 90% reported at least one change consequent to taking the course (see Table 2]. Specifically, two-thirds of the parents showed understanding to their children (a skill that involved identifying and reflecting the child's affect and its cause without further commentary), and one-third used rewards instead of punishment. Although middle and working class parents did not vary on content of their responses, the former provided more responses than the latter (mean = 1.63 ($SD=0.62$) vs. 1.14 (0.66), $t=2.06$, $P=0.05$). In addition, the quantity of responses was significantly correlated with attendance ($r = 0.53$, $P=0.003$) and homework completion ($r = 0.37$, $P=0.04$).

When asked to identify *what was most helpful* about SITIF, 90% of the parents gave one or more answers (see Table 2]. Specifically, 23.33% cited knowledge (e.g., Chinese and American cultural differences, child development) and 80% cited parenting skills. On average, middle class parents provided 2.19 responses ($SD=0.91$) and working class parents provided 1.21 responses ($SD=0.80$, $t=3.99$, df=28, $P=0.005$). Parents who attended more classes gave more responses ($r=0.37$, $P=0.04$). With regard to the most helpful skills, showing understanding and special time (where the parent devotes half an hour to interacting with the child, following the child's lead and showing understanding) were cited most often, each by 46.7% of the parents. Middle class parents were more likely to name special time as more helpful than working class parents (78.6% vs. 21.4%, using Fisher's exact test, $P=0.01$). Special time is a potentially challenging parenting method that requires the substitution of the Chinese parenting practice of guiding the child, following the child's lead continually for a recommended 30-minute period per week. Compared with working class parents, middle class parents may be more acculturated and therefore more willing to implement special time and to do so correctly. Furthermore, working class parents are more likely to be burdened with long working days and other demands that diminish their time and energy, and thus they garnered less benefit.

With regard to *what was least helpful*, the overwhelming majority of the parents responded with "nothing" or "everything was helpful." No differences were found either in quantity or in content of responses between the two socioeconomic groups, and the number of responses did not vary by engagement. Four [25%] middle class parents provided a response. Of these, three explained they were already familiar with deep breathing and child development, and one cited the skills of structure and limits. The four working class parents who responded positively (or 28.5%) to this question cited child development, and the skills of punishment (presumably meaning she would use it less now) and structure as least helpful. The remaining parent noted deep breathing was inadequate to deal with daily stress.

Finally, with regard to the ultimate objective of the intervention, that is, change in the *intergenerational relationship*, as Table 2 shows, 96.7% reported a positive change, describing it as more open, more egalitarian, and more intimate than before the intervention. Responses did not vary by either socioeconomic status/language or engagement.

Overall, after taking the SITIF course, at least 90% of the participants answered affirmatively to having changed personally, modified their parenting method, identified at least one aspect of SITIF as particularly helpful, and improved the intergenerational relationship.

Association of and Objective Mastery and Subjective Evaluation of Effectiveness

Relationship of the four domains of objective assessment (awareness/knowledge, rationale/objective of behavioral parenting skills, implementation of behavioral skills, and coping with stress) and subjective rating of SITIF's effectiveness was tested using a regression model, where the former served as the independent variable and the latter served as the dependent variable, controlling for socioeconomic status, attendance, and homework completion. The model was not significant and none of the independent and control variables significantly predicted subjective ratings of effectiveness.

Discussion

Engagement with SITIF

Measured by attendance, Chinese American parents evidenced significant engagement, attending 87% of the classes. Although middle class parents attended more classes than working class parents, the latter still attended 80% of the sessions. Variation in attendance between the two groups may be due to several reasons. Foremost, the Mandarin-speaking classes were offered at the same time and place as their children's Chinese language school. In fact, the time and location for the class were chosen in response to the parents' request. Parents found it very convenient to attend the SITIF classes while their children were attending Chinese school. In contrast, working class parents needed to make a special trip to attend SITIF classes. As their class was offered on a weekday morning, the meetings sometimes conflicted with their work schedule or other commitments. In addition, middle class parents may have been more motivated to attend SITIF than working class parents. First, they had paid a fee to attend. Second, in class and individual discussions, it was evident that they were less preoccupied with financial concerns than working class parents. As such, they were freed up to attend to their children's psychological needs and the quality of their relationship. To enhance better attendance, future SITIF classes for working class parents should be offered at a time and location of maximum convenience for them. The need for continued attendance was emphasized at an informational meeting prior to the beginning of the SITIF course, which was held for middle class parents but not working class parents. In addition, in previous research of community-based interventions, participants were given a financial incentive for attending more sessions at the time they received payment for completing the evaluation [37]. This is likely to be an effective method to boost attendance among SITIF participants.

As measured by homework completion, middle class parents demonstrated excellent engagement, as, on average, they implemented and wrote more than six of the seven sets of homework. Missing homework was primarily due to missing class when the assignment was given. Working class parents completed less homework than middle class parents. However, as they attended on average of about six classes, and thus were given five sets of homework, an average completion rate of 3.36 also supported their engagement. Modifying the expectation from writing homework to verbally reporting it reflects SITIF's sensitivity to a population less comfortable with paper–pencil tasks.

Objective Mastery of the SITIF Curriculum

Overall, using open-ended questions, parents demonstrated good mastery over the SITIF curriculum. Open-ended questions are more difficult than multiple choice or true/false questions, as parents must produce answers without relying on any hints. Across the four domains, parents showed the greatest mastery in the area of *Coping with Stress* arising in any area of their life (93.33% gave a correct response), followed by *Awareness and Knowledge* (80% gave correct responses). Performance was weaker on the two skills domains: 63.33% for *Rationale/Objective* and 56.67% for *Implementation* questions. Given the discrepancy across these four domains, it appears that devoting three sessions to behavioral parenting skills may be insufficient. More time is needed to assist solid integration. Thus, future SITIF classes should be extended to 10 sessions, with two additional classes allotted to the practice of parenting skills.

It can be noted that middle class parents surpassed working class parents in attendance, homework completion, and the number of correct responses on *Awareness/Knowledge* and *Rationale/Objective of Behavioral Parenting Skills* questions. As attendance and homework completion enhanced mastery in almost all content areas, implementation of the methods proposed above may boost attendance and enhance retention of the curriculum.

Subjective Evaluation of SITIF's Effectiveness

Using closed- and open-ended questions, both middle class and working class Chinese American parents strongly endorsed SITIF's relevance and effectiveness, giving it a 4.73 rating on a 5-point scale. Although it is plausible that responses to closed-ended subjective evaluation items may be biased due to parents' desire to please the instructor, this is less likely to be the case for the open-ended items, where parents need to specify how they were changed by participation in the SITIF class. More than 90% of the parents described how SITIF changed them personally, modified their parenting method, identified at least one helpful component of SITIF, and ultimately improved their intergenerational relationship. Working class parents provided fewer responses than middle class parents to "change in parenting method" and "what was most helpful about SITIF." As most of the responses given to the latter question also referred to parenting skills, these differences suggest that the latter retained fewer parenting skills than the former, possibly due to their lower attendance as discussed above.

Association of Objective Mastery and Subjective Evaluation of Effectiveness

Subjective evaluation of effectiveness and objective mastery of SITIF were not significantly associated. This was likely to be due to the very limited range of responses provided on the dependent variable, subjective evaluation. However, the extremely high evaluation ratings provide strong support for the utility of the SITIF intervention and its continued testing and refinement.

Study Limitations and Directions for Future Research

The current study demonstrated SITIF's effectiveness in strengthening the intergenerational relationship with a diverse group of Chinese American immigrant parents. Extending the SITIF course to 10 sessions and improving attendance among working class parents using methods proposed above may further enhance its effectiveness. In future research, a randomized, controlled design should be used to rule out other potential contributions to postintervention changes. The study suffers from the absence of baseline data on parenting and the intergenerational relationship. As reported previously, baseline data were collected using standardized, quantitative measures from middle class parents and demonstrated significant pre–post intervention improvement in parenting efficacy and intergenerational relationship [30, 31]. However, because working class parents expressed significant difficulties responding to the questions despite individualized assistance and verbal administration, these were discarded. Future research needs to utilize measures with simpler wordings that reflect Chinese colloquial expressions. In addition, due to the small sample size, it was not possible to assess potential variation by demographic characteristics other than socioeconomic status. This should be addressed in future research. Fathers comprised only 16.7% of the current sample; future research should target more fathers. Furthermore, assessing change in the target child and/or the child's view of the intergenerational relationship would further support SITIF's effectiveness. Future studies should also assess the long-term effects of SITIF, which may suggest the need for booster sessions to maintain its effect. Finally, they should empirically test SITIF's effectiveness in non-Chinese immigrant populations. Of particular interest are Latino Americans, who comprise the largest immigrant group in the United States. In spite of these limitations, the study makes a significant contribution to the literature on immigrant families by demonstrating the utility of the newly developed SITIF curriculum in enhancing parenting effectiveness and intergenerational intimacy among a diverse group of Chinese American immigrant parents.

References

1. Sluzki C. Migration and family conflict. Fam Process 1979;18:379–390.
2. Drachman D, Kwon-Ahn YH, Paulino A. Migration and resettlement experiences of Dominican and Korean families. Fam Soc 1996;December: 626–638.
3. Garcia Coll CT, Meyer EC, Brillon L. Ethnic and minority parenting. In: Bornstein MY, ed. *Handbook of Parenting: Biology and Ecology of Parenting*, vol. 2. Mawhaw, NJ: Lawrence Erlbaum, 1995:189–210.
4. Kibria N. *Family Tightrope: The Changing Lives of Vietnamese Americans*. Princeton, NJ: Princeton University Press, 1993.
5. Kwak K. Adolescents and their parents: A review of intergenerational family relations for immigrant and non-immigrant families. Hum Dev 2003;46:115–136.
6. Lee RM, Choe J, Kim G, Ngo V. Construction of the Asian American Family Conflicts Scale. J Couns Psychol 2000;47:211–222.
7. Portes A, Rumbaut RG, *Immigrant America: A Portrait*, 2nd ed. Berkeley: University of California Press, 1996.
8. Ying Y, Chao C. Intergenerational relationship in Iu Mien American families. Amerasia J 1996;22:47–64.
9. Ying Y, Han M. The longitudinal effect of intergenerational gap in acculturation on conflict and mental health in Southeast Asian American adolescents. Am J Orthopsychiatry 2007; 77:61–66.

10. Zhou M, Bankston CL III. *Growing up American: How Vietnamese Children Adapt to Life in the United States.* New York: Russell Sage Foundation, 1998.
11. Buki LP, Ma T, Strom RD, Strom SK. Chinese immigrant mothers of adolescents: Self-perceptions of acculturation effects on parenting. Cultur Divers Ethnic Minor Psychol 2003;9:127–140.
12. Ying Y, Lee PA, & Tsai JL. Psychometric Properties of the Intergenerational Congruence in Immigrant Families: Child Scale in Chinese Americans. J Comp Fam Stud 2004;35: 91–103.
13. Ying Y, Tracy L. Psychometric properties of the intergenerational congruence in immigrant families – parent scale in Chinese Americans. Soc Work Res 2004;28:56–62.
14. Ho DY. Relational orientation in Asian social psychology. In: Kim U, Berry JW, eds. *Indigenous Psychologies: Research and Experience in Cultural Context.* Newbury Park, CA: Sage Publications, 1993:240–259.
15. Greenberger E, Chen C. Perceived family relationships and depressed mood in early and late adolescence: A comparison of European and Asian Americans. Dev Psychol 1996;32:707–716.
16. Kurtines WM, Miranda L. Differences in self and family role perception among acculturating Cuban American college students. Int J Intercult Relat 1980;4:167–184.
17. Ying Y, Lee PA, Tsai JL, Lee YJ, Tsang M. Relationship of young Chinese American adults with their parents: Variation by migratory status and cultural orientation. Am J Orthopsychiatry 2001;71:342–349.
18. Chung RG. Gender, ethnicity, and acculturation in intergenerational conflict of Asian American college students. Cultur Divers Ethnic Minor Psychol 2001;7: 376–386.
19. Rumbaut RG. The crucible within: Ethnic identity, self-esteem, and segmented assimilation among children of immigrants. In: Portes A, ed. *The New Second Generation.* New York: Russell Sage Foundation, 1996:119–170.
20. Portes A, Zhou M. The new second generation: Segmented assimilation and its variants. Ann Am Acad Pol Soc Sci 1993;530:74–96.
21. Waters MC. Ethnic and racial identities of second generation Black immigrants in New York City. Int Migr Rev 1994;28:795–820.
22. Zhou M. Growing up American: The challenge confronting immigrant children and children of immigrants. Annu Rev Sociol 1997;23:63–95.
23. Szapocznik J, Kurtines W, Santisteban DA, Pantin H, Scopetta M, Mancilla Y, et al. The evolution of structural ecosystemic theory for working with Latino families. In: Garcia JG, Zea MC, eds. *Psychological Interventions and Research with Latino Populations*, Boston: Allyn and Bacon, 1997:160–190.
24. US Census Bureau. U.S. Census Bureau Fact and Features: Asian Pacific American Heritage Month: May 2003, 2003. Available at http://www.census.gov/Press-Release/www/2003/cb03ff06.html.
25. Hendricks T. Foreign-born residents on rise, Census reports. San Francisco Chronicle June 5 2002:A17.
26. Capps R, Fix M, Ost J, Reardon-Anderson J, Passel JS. *The Health and Well-Being of Young Children of Immigrants.* Washington, DC: Urban Institute, 2004.
27. Sandoval MC, De La Roza M. Cultural perspectives for serving the Hispanic client. In: Lefley HP, Pedersen PB, eds. *Cross-Cultural Training for Mental Health Professionals.* Springfield, IL: Charles C. Thomas, 1986:151–160.
28. Falicov CJ. Mexican families. In: McGoldrick M, Pearce, JK, Giordano J. eds. *Ethnicity and the Family.* New York: Guilford Press, 1982:134–153.
29. Ying Y, Coombs M, Lee PA. Family intergenerational relationship of Asian American adolescents. Cultur Divers Ethnic Minor Psychol 1999;5:350–363.
30. Ying Y. An educational program for families on intergenerational conflict. In: Kramer E, Ivey S, Ying Y. eds. *Immigrant Women's Health: Problems and Solutions.* San Francisco: Jossey-Bass, 1999:282–294.

31. Ying Y. Strengthening intergenerational/intercultural ties in migrant families: A new intervention for parents. J Community Psychol 1999a;27:89–96.
32. Szapocznik J, Truss C. Intergenerational sources of role conflict in Cuban mothers. In: Monteil M, ed. *Hispanic Families: Critical Issues for Policy and Programs in Human Services*, Washington, DC: National Coalition of Hispanic Mental Health and Human Services Organizations, 1978:41–65.
33. Adler P, Ovando C, Hocevar D. Familiar correlates of gang membership: An exploratory study. Hisp J Behav Sci 1984;6:65–76.
34. Aldwin C, Greenberger E. Cultural differences in predictors of depression. Am J Community Psychol 1987;15:789–813.
35. Hernandez-Guzman L, Sanchez-Sosa JJ. Parent-child interactions predict anxiety in Mexican adolescents. Adolescence 1996;31:953–963.
36. Bandura A. *Social Learning Theory*. Englewood Cliffs, NJ: Prentice-Hall, 1977.
37. Munoz RF, Ying Y. *The Prevention of Depression: Research and Practice*. Baltimore: Johns Hopkins University Press, 2002.
38. Lum D. *Culturally Competent Practice*. Pacific Grove, CA: Brooks/Cole, 1999.
39. Zayas LH, Torres LR, Malcolm J, DesRosiers FS. Clinicians' definitions of ethnic sensitive therapy. Prof Psychol Res Pr 1996;27:78–82.
40. Sue S, Zane NW. The role of culture and cultural techniques in psychotherapy: A critique and reformulation. Am Psychol 1987;42:37–45.
41. Sue S, Fujino D, Hu L, Takeuchi D, Zane N. Community mental health services for ethnic minority groups: A test of the cultural responsiveness hypothesis. J Consult Clin Psychol 1991;59:533–540.
42. Snowden L, Cheung F. Use of inpatient mental health services by members of ethnic minority groups. Am Psychol 1990;45:347–355.
43. Guerney BG Jr. Filial therapy: Description and rationale. J Consult Psychol 1964;28:303–310.
44. Guerney L. *The Parenting Skills Manual: Leader's Manual*. State College, PA: IDEALS 1987.
45. Greenbaum L, Holmes IH. The use of folktales in social work practice. Soc Casework 1983:414–418.
46. US Census Bureau. The foreign-born population in the United States: March 2002. Washington, DC: U.S. Department of Commerce, 2003a:P20–P539.
47. Yu E, Zhang M. Translation of instruments: Procedures, issues, and dilemmas. In: Liu, WT, ed. *A Decade Review of Mental Health Research, Training, and Services*. Chicago: Pacific/Asian American Mental Health Research Center, 1987:101–107.
48. Rubin A, Babbie ER. *Research Methods for Social Work*, 5th ed. Belmont, CA: Brooks/Cole, 2005.
49. Rounsaville BJ, Carroll KM, Onken LS. A stage model of behavioral therapies research: Getting started and moving from stage 1. Clin Psychol 2001;2:134–142.

Acculturation: Recommendations for Future Research

Richard M. Suinn

Abstract In this chapter, future directions in acculturation research and design are suggested which could provide valuable new insights and knowledge. Topics discussed include the importance of subject-selection procedures (ranging from individual characteristics to group commonalities), various measurement issues (such as instrumentation and scoring methods), and research design procedures (including discussion of complexities in design).

Keywords Acculturation research · Acculturation research design · Individual differences · Research directions · Acculturation measurement

Contents

Summarization of Previous Chapters	65
Considerations for Future Research	66
Research Populations and Subject Selection	67
Measurement Procedure Issues	71
General Research Design Considerations	73
Summary	74
References	74

Summarization of Previous Chapters

The first three chapters in this volume present diverse perspectives regarding contemporary research on acculturation. The chapter by Suinn focuses on acculturation, defined as a process that can occur when two or more cultures interact together. Conducting research on acculturation requires the availability of standard measurement instruments. Several such research measures are identified in this chapter along with the rationale and characteristics of each

R.M. Suinn (✉)
Department of Psychology, Colorado State University, Fort Collins, CO 80523, USA
e-mail: suinn@lamar.colostate.edu

(the instruments themselves appear in Appendix). The chapter then provides a comprehensive review of research demonstrating the influence of acculturation on physical health, mental health, school performance, choice of careers, and attitudes toward counseling and therapy. These findings provide convincing support for the conclusion that the level of acculturation has a crucial role in nearly every facet of the lives of Asian Americans and their families.

The chapter by Kim extends the focus by elaborating on the concepts of acculturation and enculturation. Here Kim defines acculturation as the process of adapting to the norms of the US culture, and enculturation as the process of becoming socialized into and maintaining the norms of the Asian culture. Therefore, whereas chapter 1 summarizes existing research on acculturation, chapter 2 expounds by focusing more on enculturation. Using the concept of enculturation, Kim identifies intergenerational conflict as an outcome of a parent who remains high in enculturation but low in acculturation levels and a child who is high in acculturation and low in enculturation levels. A summary of selected research on intergenerational conflict is provided, leading to the description of Kim's own study on the role of cognitive flexibility and intergenerational conflict. His research design illustrates how sensitivity to the ethnic population can be integrated into the study's procedures. For example, his study highlights the importance of considering a variety of community access points: Korean cultural awareness groups, Korean churches, the Educational Opportunity Program, and the Resource Center for Sexual and Gender Diversity. Kim also recognized the limitations of the English-only instruments. Hence, for those with limited English proficiency, instruments were in Korean using the forward–back translation method.

In the chapter by Ying, the significant influence of intergenerational conflict is further discussed. While Kim's research studies the role of a mediating variable on family conflict (observational study), Ying focuses on an intervention to prevent such conflict (experimental study). Details of Ying's research on a community-based intervention program are provided. Of interest is the use of design procedures that enhanced the sensitivity of the research to the needs of the participants. For instance, there was a shared venue for data collection and intervention, which was particularly convenient for the participants. This highlights the importance of thoughtful access points. In addition, both written and oral homework were accepted, which helped to retain participants in the study. Finally, the language selected for the intervention was matched to the participants' preference and primary language use. This was an additional procedure that aided in successful measurement.

Considerations for Future Research

As seen in these first three chapters, there exists a foundation of scholarly studies that establish not only the relevance but also the importance of studying acculturation status as a variable. These studies need to now be followed by further work if the field is to reach maturity and contribute further insights about Asian Americans. To achieve such goals, certain design issues need to be addressed. The following sections suggest directions for the refinement of future research on acculturation, including attention to how participant groups are defined and clustered, which measurement procedures are selected, and how the research itself is designed and implemented.

Research Populations and Subject Selection

Identifying Study Populations by Groups

Nearly all prior research has been based on various ethnic groups in which data are combined as representing "Asians" or "Asian Americans." Many are from the most accessible populations such as college students. Sample sizes tend to be reasonably large, with some surveys being large enough to be considered as representative samples of certain populations. However, future research might benefit from distinguishing among groups and focusing on specifics such as ethnicity and age and widening the scope of the types of persons studied.

Identification by group: Ethnic identities. Clearly, more attention needs to be paid to separating out data from various ethnic Asian American populations into smaller groupings, of which there are an estimated 60 separate "Asian" subgroups. For instance, the term "Asian" refers to such varied subgroups as Koreans, Asian Indians, Filipinos, and Hmong. However, despite the use of a single label, not all "Asian" groups are alike. Kim et al. [1] examined data on 570 Chinese, Filipino, Korean, and Japanese American college students using the Asian Values Scale (AVS) [2]. This scale covers six value dimensions characterizing Asian cultures: collectivism, conformity to norms, emotional self-control, family recognition through achievement, filial piety, and humility. Results confirmed that significant differences in adherence to these values do exist when the different Asian groups were compared. Ying and her colleagues [3, 4] examined the characteristics of "Southeast Asians," another grouping of Asians often joined together in research. Ying's sample included Hmong, Vietnamese, and Cambodians refugees. Results showed that differences in cultural identity existed among these three groups. The most traditional were the Hmong and the least traditional were the Vietnamese, with the Cambodians in between. This confirms that despite coming from the same geographic area, Southeast Asians from different ethnic groups cannot be viewed as identical to one another. It is noteworthy that in Ying's follow-up study, different results were found [5]. The sample included Hmong, Vietnamese, and Cambodian college students who were either American-born or early-arriving (by age 5 years). Cultural orientation was again assessed and compared across groups. Unlike the older refugee samples, no significant differences were found among the groups on the level of cultural orientation. Ultimately, the acculturation experience dissipated differences that might have existed in the parental generations.

Burlew [6] emphasized recognition of the diversity within subgroupings (intraethnic differences). By using such an approach, important within-group variation may be identified. For instance, a study might restrict its group to being a study of "Japanese," but caution is needed before generalizing to all Japanese. The research of Marmot et al. [7] found differences in coronary heart disease depending on whether the Japanese in the study were from Japan, Hawaii, or California. Williams et al. [8] studied Japanese Americans in Hawaii. Although some studies report low acculturation to be associated with acculturation stress, which in turn is associated with psychological symptoms, Williams et al. [8] found the reverse. In their sample, higher Japanese values, activities, and lifestyle were associated with lower depressive symptoms. Is this a finding unique to Japanese American populations, or perhaps even restricted to Japanese American populations living in Hawaii? Despite the existence of some commonalities among Asian populations, this one study demonstrates that clustering groups together as "Asians" or even as "Japanese" can easily overlook importance differences.

Identification by group: Immigrant status. Another distinction can be made in distinguishing between refugee and non-refugee immigrants [9]. Refugees come from a background of trauma or political stress and may be viewed as escaping from their home country; immigrants may be viewed as seeking further benefits as they approach the new country [10, 11]. Pin-Riebe et al. [12] identified severe experiences of trauma among refugees: 60% of Cambodians and 48% of Vietnamese reported being robbed, raped, or tortured during their escape from their country. Furthermore, 95% experienced death of at least one member of their family from "unnatural causes." For immigrants, acculturative stress may be present, as they have lost property and may be entering low-status employment and living conditions. Among the elderly, they might for the first time face the loss of status or veneration for their wisdom and age [13].

In future research regarding immigrants' or refugees' acculturation process, contextual and environmental factors may prove important. For instance, it may be revealing to examine the role served by the places chosen for settlement. Of relevance might be the characteristics of the new residency; for example, the size of the town or city, the level of diversity within their new area of residence, the climate of tolerance, or the availability of social support systems. These factors might themselves be important influences.

Identification by group: Families. A variety of studies have looked at families, such as those involving intergenerational differences in acculturation status. Even within families, there can be different distinctions deserving of investigation. For example, there are families with role reversals following immigration, where the traditional salary earning "head of the family" might shift. In addition, the so-called "astronaut families" or families separated for long periods may be presented with a different family dynamic when the family is together again [14, 15]. Families may also be distinguished based on socioeconomic status. In Ying's study in this volume, socioeconomic differences were associated with geographic differences as well as language preference. For example, the middle class group came from Taiwan and preferred Mandarin, while the working class came from China and preferred Cantonese. Therefore, it would be important to consider differences among families and within families when considering subject selection.

Identifying Study Populations by Individual Characteristics

Identification by individual characteristics: Personality. Studies on acculturation might benefit from giving attention to the personal characteristics of individuals, as these might interact with the influence of acculturation. As cited in Kim's earlier chapter, Ahn et al. [16] and Harrison et al. [17] have studied cognitive flexibility. Cognitive flexibility involves awareness that options and alternatives are available in any situation; it also includes the willingness and competence to adapt to any given situation [18]. Ahn et al. found that increased cognitive flexibility was associated with decreased intergenerational conflict in the area of dating and marriage [16].

Chang [19] compared Asian Americans with European Americans to identify the possible influence of optimism/pessimism and positive/negative affectivity on psychological stress and symptoms. Although acculturation status was not studied, results demonstrated differential effects of these personality variables on stress and symptoms. Therefore, it is possible that adding person-specific characteristics as a variable, such as cognitive flexibility or optimism/pessimism, to studies on acculturation might also reveal new insights. These individual characteristics might serve as protective factors from acculturative stress, and thus warrant further investigation. Among those worthy of attention include cognitive flexibility, facility in acquiring languages, self-esteem, optimism/pessimism, positive/negative affectivity, coping characteristics, and possibly spirituality [20–28]

Identification by individual characteristics: Language. Skill in the language of the host country is sometimes viewed as useful in coping and reducing the stress of the acculturation process [23, 29, 30]. However, Unger et al. [31] actually concluded that English language proficiency could be a "risk factor" for smoking initiation. One hypothesis is that English proficiency enables an increase in exposure to and awareness of pro-tobacco media messages. Other studies have also reported inconsistent findings regarding language effects. Kennedy and Park [32] reported that, for Asian American middle-school students, speaking a language other than English in the home was positively related to course grades. However, Mouw and Xie [33] found no positive effects of bilingualism, and concluded that the occasional effects are temporary. As language is often used as an index of acculturation, more research on language skills as a variable might prove useful

Identification by individual characteristics: Developmental age. Developmental age of the individual at the time of immigration is another factor deserving of study [34–36]. Hwang et al. [37] studied the impact of age of immigration, using six developmental periods: childhood, adolescence, young adulthood,

adulthood, middle adulthood, and later adulthood. They found that lower acculturation status in addition to the age of immigration was predictive of depression. More specifically, the risk for depression decreased 6% for every 1-year increase in age at immigration. Thus, they conclude "those who immigrate at younger ages evidence greater overall risk for depression onset than those who immigrate at later ages" (p. 22).

Identification by individual characteristics: Gender. Gender is another individual characteristic that should be separated out as a study variable. Chung et al. [38] reported that female Vietnamese immigrants acculturated more rapidly than male Vietnamese immigrants. Hofstetter et al. [39] also found gender differences in their study of Koreans living in California. Higher rates of smoking were associated for men with lower acculturation status, but with higher acculturation status for women. In addition, while Tang and Dion [40] argued that Chinese men face more acculturation challenges than Chinese women, Furnham and Shiekh [41] concluded that female Asian immigrants tend to have more severe mental health symptoms than male immigrant counterparts. With regard to intergenerational conflicts between parents and children, Chung [42] found differences between adolescent females and males. Females experienced greater conflicts about dating and marriage issues than males. In the earlier chapters of this volume, both Kim and Ying state that there may have been important information gleaned if responses from both fathers and mothers were collected. More research is needed that may elucidate important gender differences.

Identification by individual characteristics: Multiracial heritage. Another personal characteristic that may warrant attention in acculturation research is that of multiracial heritage. Choi et al. [43] compared data on African-, Asian-, and European American youths with multiracial youths in school in Seattle. There were 25 combinations of multiracial groupings. The largest multiracial group was those of African American/Native American heritage (22.7% of 454 multiracial participants), with the second largest being the European/Asian American combination (11.5%, 41). For analyses, all multiracial participants were combined. Controlling for age, gender, and income status, the multiracial adolescents were more likely to have smoked or used alcohol. Marijuana, crack, or cocaine use and violent behaviors were more characteristic of the multiracial youths than the Asian American youths. Williams et al. [8] analyzed results on Japanese and part-Japanese adolescents in Hawaii. The Japanese American students scored higher on Japanese identity than the multiracial adolescents, suggesting that the part-Japanese students found it difficult to identify with the Japanese culture. Furthermore, the Japanese American adolescents scored lower on depression symptoms than the part-Japanese counterparts. Finally, relevant to gender issues, part-Japanese females scored higher on the practice of Japanese lifestyle than part-Japanese males. Thus, for mixed-heritage persons, the acculturation/enculturation processes and identity development process are particularly complex.

Measurement Procedure Issues

Instrumentation. It is important to recognize that "acculturation status" reported in research is operationally defined in various ways. As the acculturation process is considered to involve changes resulting from exposure to another culture over time, then length of time in the host country may be one definition. However, there has been more attention given to measurements defining acculturation either by behaviors or by values. Kim et al. [44] identified two separate factors in examining the AVS versus the Suinn-Lew Asian Self-Identity Acculturation Scale (SL-ASIA), one corresponding to values and the other corresponding to behaviors. The correlation between the Asian values acculturation scale and the behavioral acculturation scale was 0.15. This demonstrates that the two scales are measuring different constructs. Thus, differing formal measures of acculturation are available. But behaviorally focused measurements and values-focused measurements are not necessarily equally successful in predicting specific outcome variables. The point is that research findings may differ because different definitions/measures of acculturation were used; for example, acculturation defined by the length of residence or by different standardized instruments. This will be made clear in the next section.

Behavioral acculturation versus values acculturation. The previously mentioned discussion about behaviors versus values measures deserves further elaboration. Although both have been accepted as appropriate reflections of acculturation, there is some value in studying each independently and defining what appropriate uses are for each [45]. It has been hypothesized that the acculturation process involving changes in cultural behaviors might occur at a faster pace than changes in the individual's commitment to cultural values [46, 47]. This alone would imply that a study using a behaviorally focused scale might reveal results very different than if a values-focused scale were used. Shim [48] found that a values measure of acculturation status was a better predictor of cultural adjustment among Korean Americans than a behavioral measure. On the other hand, Choo [49] reported that a behavioral measure of acculturation status was a better predictor of family adjustment than a values measure among Asian Americans.

Suinn [50] has also suggested that the accuracy of relying on values-focused indices or behaviorally focused indices to predict outcomes might depend on the situation or context being predicted. For example, consider an attempt to predict behaviors of an adolescent occurring in the context of the individual being surrounded by Western peers: a behaviorally focused measure of acculturation might prove more accurate than a values-focused scale. On the other hand, consider an attempt to predict the behavior of an Asian selecting a spouse when first-generation parents are present. A values-focused measure of acculturation might be more accurate here than a behaviorally focused scale. Even within instruments measuring values, scores on different values have been found to differ in the variables these values predict. Park and Kim [51] used the Asian American Values Scale – Multidimensional [52], which provides scores on five Asian culture values: emotional control, humility, collectivism, conformity to norms, and family recognition through achievement. They found that different values were associated with different communication styles. For instance, scores on collectivism values were positively associated with a contentious or challenging communication style, but humility was negatively associated with this style of communicating. In effect, specific types of values and behaviors and their appropriate corresponding scales may be critical to consider when determining study design.

Before leaving the topic of measurement instruments, attention should be called to Kim's reference in this volume to two more dimensions: knowledge and identity as aspects of acculturation. Knowledge is measured by assessing the person's knowledge of culture-specific information, such as the meaning of cultural holidays or activities. Identity is measured by assessing the individual's self-statement about personal ethnic identity. In the same way that behavioral measures may have a different significance from values measures in acculturation research, the same may hold true for the concepts of knowledge or identity [53]. As an illustration of the complexity in the area of research on Asian Americans, Yoo and Lee [54] explored the question of whether ethnic identity buffers or exacerbates experiences of racism. They discovered that Asian American students strongly identified with their ethnicity experienced high positive emotions after experiencing a single racism incident, while students with low identification reported lower positive emotions following such an experience. On the other hand, for multiple incidents of racism, the results were reversed. There was also a complex interaction effect among ethnic identity (high or low), racism (single or multiple), and immigration status (immigrant or US born). Therefore, future research assessing these types of dimensions might uncover more data regarding acculturation.

Identifying the phase of acculturation. Another topic deserving attention in acculturation research is the identification of the "interim" phase of the acculturation process; this is the phase where the acculturation process is still ongoing and not yet complete. Studies that use length of time in the host country come the closest to recognizing this idea (e.g., see Chen et al. [55]). With this as a study variable, new hypotheses could be explored. For instance, does the level of acculturative stress vary as a function of time in the host country? After a lengthy residence in the host country, does an immigrant's failure to acquire behavioral competency (such as language) contribute to higher stress levels? How does length of residence in the host country affect evaluations from Western observers based on their anticipation about the immigrant's expected progress?After extensive residence in the host country, would a person who fails to integrate or assimilate be more subject to racism or discrimination?Are there differences in outcomes for a person who alternates years of residency in two societies?

Orthogonal scoring. It is important to assess participants' status regarding attitudes, behaviors, and values of the country of origin as well as assessing their status regarding the host country. As stated earlier, an individual may have a combination of attitudes toward their host country and country of origin. They may be as follows: (1) high in commitment to the host country and low in commitment to the country of origin; (2) low in commitment to the host country but high in commitment to the country of origin; (3) high in commitment to the host country and high in commitment to the country of origin; or (4) low in commitment to the host country and low in commitment to the country of origin. Herskovitz [56] first offered the term "enculturation" to be the process of socialization to the norms of one's indigenous culture. Kim and Abreu [57] defined acculturation as the process of adapting to the norms of the dominant group (i.e., European American) and enculturation as the process of retaining the norms of the indigenous group (e.g., Asian American). As explained in Suinn's prior chapter in this volume, instruments recognizing this distinction are referred to as orthogonal scales. From such a distinction comes the development of measures such as the European American Values Scale for Asian Americans, the AVS and the Asian American Multidimensional Acculturation Scale. Similarly, Abe-Kim et al. [58] developed a scoring scheme for the SL-ASIA that permitted scores for Asian orientation level, European American orientation level, and bicultural orientation level. Mallinckrodt et al. [59] used a scoring procedure for the SL-ASIA that provides two independent scores: Traditional Culture Identification (TCI) index and Western Cultural Identification (WCI) index. The concepts of the "marginalized" person or the "bicultural" person are derived from this approach. Kim et al. [60] confirmed that marginalized persons were more vulnerable to depression. LaFromboise et al. [61] have concluded that bicultural competency enables better psychological and physical health and facilitates performance in academic and vocational endeavors. In support of this, Nguyen et al, [62] reported that bicultural Vietnamese youth had more positive family relationships and higher self-esteem (in Kim, 26).

General Research Design Considerations

Over the span of research on acculturation, studies have shifted from examining single variables to complex variables. Earlier studies straightforwardly studied the association between acculturation level and a specific outcome, firming up the conclusion that acculturation is a significant factor. More complex research designs have become possible along with more sophisticated statistical analyses to examine relationships among several variables [63]. Research now includes analyses such as structural equation modeling [8], structural invariance analysis [64], logistic regression analysis [65], proportional hazards modeling [37], and hierarchical regression analysis [36, 66].

Mediating variables. With the availability of more complex research designs and statistical techniques, research can continue to examine multiple variables that mediate between acculturation status and outcomes. Examples of mediator variables that interact with acculturation status can be found in studies formulating models of pathways. For instance, low Western identity among youth combined with symptoms of general parent/child conflicts is predictive of adolescent suicide [65]. Similarly, high Asian identity status among South Asian Americans tends to be associated with higher occupational self-efficacy about traditional careers, which in turn is predictive of career choice [67]. In addition, highly Westernized adolescents are vulnerable to alcohol binge drinking when exposed to peer influence [68]. Furthermore, for adolescents with low parental attachment, the odds of alcohol use are 11 times greater in the more highly acculturated group than in the less acculturated group [69]. Finally, acculturation discrepancy between youths and parents is associated with youth violence but as mediated by the presence of delinquent peers [70]. Such studies add more detailed understanding of the conditions or pathways whereby acculturation affects diverse life outcomes.

Summary

There is no question that acculturation is a relevant and an important topic for study regarding Asian Americans and their families. The research and reviews described in the initial three chapters provide convincing evidence. However, there are as many new questions raised by these studies as are answered. The current chapter focuses on various recommendations for future research. Such recommendations include various ways of identifying the group to be sampled, type of individual characteristics deserving of study, measurement issues needing to be addressed, and possible research designs that might be considered. The foundation is here; the topic is deserving; the future is waiting.

References

1. Kim B, Yang P, Atkinson D, Wolfe M, Hong S. Cultural value similarities and differences among Asian American ethnic groups. Cultur Divers Ethnic Minor Psychol 2001;7: 343–361.
2. Kim B, Atkinson D. Yang P. The Asian Values Scale (AVS) Development, factor analysis, validation, and reliability. J Couns Psychol 1999;46:342–352.
3. Ying Y, Akutsu P. Psychological adjustment of Southeast Asian refugees: The contribution of sense of coherence. J Community Psychol 1997;25:125–139.
4. Ying Y, Akutsu P, Zhang, X, Huang L. Psychological dysfunction in Southeast Asian refugees as mediated by sense of coherence. Am J Community Psychol 1997;25:839–859.
5. Ying Y, Han M. Cultural orientation in Southeast Asian American young adults. Cultur Divers Ethnic Minor Psychol 2008;14:29–37.
6. Burlew A. Research with ethnic minorities. Conceptual, methodological, and analytic issues. In Bernal G, Trimble J, Burlew A, Leong F. eds. *Handbook of Racial and Ethnic Minority Psychology*. Thousand Oaks, CA: Sage, 2003:179–197.
7. Marmot M, Syme S, Kagan A, Kato H, Cohen J, Belsky J. Epidemiologic studies of coronary heart disease and stroke in Japanese men living in Japan, Hawaii and California: prevalence of coronary and hypertensive heart disease and associated risk factors. Am J Epidemiol 1975;102:514–525.

8. Williams J, Else I. Hishinuma E, Goebert D, Chang J, Andrade N, Nishimura, S. A confirmatory model for depression among Japanese American and part-Japanese American adolescents. Cultur Divers Ethnic Minor Psychol 2005;11:41–56.
9. Chung R, Bemak F. Asian immigrants and refugees. In Leong, F, Inman A, Ebreo A, Yang L, Kinoshita K, Fu M. eds. *Handbook of Asian-American Psychology*, 2nd ed. Thousand Oaks, CA: Sage 2006:227–243.
10. Marshall G, Schell T, Elliott M, Berthold S, Chun, C. Mental health of Cambodian refugees 2 decades after resettlement in the United States. JAMA 2005;294:571–579.
11. Foster R. When immigration is trauma: Guidelines for the individual and family clinician. Am J Orthopsychiatry 2001;71:153–170.
12. Pin-Riebe S, Connell J, Doung S, Pham T, Tran, H. Along the journey: Perspectives on working with Southeast Asian elderly. Paper presented at the University of Massachusetts at Boston's Culture, Mental Health, and Aging Conference, Boston, MA. 1999.
13. Gerber L, Nguyen Q, Bounkeu P. Working with Southeast Asian people who have migrated to the United States. In Nader K, Dubrow N, Stamm B. eds. Honoring Differences: Cultural Issues in the Treatment of Trauma and Loss. Philadelphia: Brunner/Mazel, 1999:98–118.
14. Alaggia R, Chau S, Tsang K. Astronaut Asian families: Impact of migration on family structure from the perspective of the youth J Soc Work Res Eval 2001;2:295–306.
15. Aye A, Guerin B. Astronaut families: A review of their characteristics, impact on families and implications for practice in New Zealand. N Z J Psychol 2001;30:9–15.
16. Ahn, AJ, Kim BSK, Park YS (in press). Asian cultural values gap, cognitive flexibility, coping strategies, and child–parent conflict among Korean Americans. Cultur Divers Ethnic Minor Psychol.
17. Harrison, AO, Wilson, MN, Pine, CJ, Chan, SQ. Family ecologies of ethnic minority children. Child Dev 1990; 60: 347–362.
18. Martin, MM, Rubin, RB. A new measure of cognitive flexibility. Psychol Rep 1995; 76, 623–626.
19. Chang E. Cultural differences in psychological distress in Asian and Caucasian American college students: Examining the role of cognitive and affective concomitants. J Couns Psychol 2002;49,:47–59.
20. Chang H. Ng, K. The perception of resiliency mechanisms in Chinese American families: Implications for family therapy. Fam Ther 2002;29:89–100.
21. Dion K, Dion K, Pak A. Personality-based hardiness as a buffer for discrimination-related stress in members of Toronto's Chinese community. Can J Behav Sci 1992;24:517–536.
22. Diwan S, Jonnalagadda S, Balaswamy S. Resources Predicting Positive and Negative Affect During the Experience of Stress: A Study of Older Asian Indian Immigrants in the United States. Gerontol 2004;44:605–614.
23. Kang S. Measurement of acculturation, scale formats, and language competence: Their Implications for Adjustment. J Cross Cult Psychol 2006;37: 669–693.
24. Kim B, Omizo M. Asian and European American cultural values, collective self-esteem, acculturative stress, cognitive flexibility, and general self-efficacy among Asian American college students. J Couns Psychol 2005;52:412–419.
25. Lee R. Resilience against discrimination: ethnic identity and other-group orientation as protective factors for Korean Americans. J Couns Psychol 2005;52:36–44.
26. Takakura M, Sakihara S. Psychosocial correlates of depressive symptoms among Japanese high school students. J Adolesc Health;28:82–89.
27. Tsai J, Ying Y, Lee P. Cultural predictors of self-esteem: A study of Chinese American female and male young adults. Cultur Divers Ethnic Minor Psychol 2001;7:284–297.
28. Goldston D, Molock S, Whitbeck L, Murakami J, Zayas L, Hall G. Cultural considerations in adolescent suicide prevention and psychosocial treatment Am Psychol 2008;63:14–31.
29. Yeh C, Kim A, Pituc S, Atkins M. Poverty, loss and resilience: The story of Chinese immigrant youth. J Couns Psychol. 2008;55:34–48.

30. Lee J, Koeske G, Sales E. Social support buffering of acculturative stress: a study of mental health symptoms among Korean international students. Int J Intercult Rel 2004:28:399–414.
31. Unger J, Cruz T, Rohrbach L, Ribisi K, Baezconde-Garbanati L, Chen X, Trinidad, D, Johnson C. English language use as a risk actor for smoking initiation among Hispanic and Asian American adolescents: Evidence for mediation by tobacco-related believes and social norms. Health Psychol 2000; 19:403–410.
32. Kennedy E, Park H. Home language as a predictor of academic achievement: A comparative study of Mexican- and Asian-American youth. J Res Dev Educ 1994;27:188–194.
33. Mouw T, Xie Y. Bilingualism and the academic achievement of first- and second-generation Asian Americans: Accommodation with or without assimilation? Am Sociol Rev 1999;64:232–252.
34. Alegria M, Mulvaney-Day N, Torres M, Polo A, Cao Z, Canino G. Prevalence of psychiatric disorders across Latino subgroups in the United States. Am J Public Health 2007;97:1–8.
35. Angel, J., & Angel, R. Age at migration, social connections, and well-being among elderly Hispanics. J Aging Health 1992;4:480–499.
36. Yeh C. Age, acculturatioin, cultural adjustment, and mental health symptoms of Chinese, Korean, and Japanese immigrant youths. Cultur Divers Ethnic Minor Psychol 2003;9:34–48.
37. Hwang W, Chun C, Takeuchi D, Myers H, Siddarth P. Age of First onset major depression in Chinese Americans. Cultur Divers Ethnic Minor Psychol 2005;11:16–27.
38. Chung R, Bemak F, Wong S. Social support and acculturation: Implications for mental health counseling. J Ment Health Couns 2000;22:150–161.
39. Hofstetter C, Hovell M, Lee J, Zakarian J, Park H, Paik H, Irvin V. Tobacco use and acculturation among Californians of Korean descent: A behavioral epidemiological analysis. Nicotine Tob Res 2004;6:481–489.
40. Tang T, Dion K. Gender and acculturation in relation to traditionalism: Perceptions of self and parents among Chinese students. Sex Roles 1999;41:17–29
41. Furnham A, Shiekh S. Gender, generational and social support correlates of mental health in Asian immigrants. Int J Soc Psychiatry 1993;9:22–33.
42. Chung R. Gender, ethnicity, and acculturation in intergenerational conflict of Asian American college students. Cult Divers Ethn Minor Psychol 2001;7:376–86.
43. Choi Y, Harachi T, Gillmore M, Catalana R. Are multiracial adolescents at greater risk? Comparisons of rates, patterns, and correlates of substance use and violence between monoracial and multiracial adolescents. Am J Orthopsychiatry 2006;76:86–97.19.
44. Kim B, Atkinson D, Yang P. The Asian Values Scale: Development, factor analysis, validation, and reliability. J Couns Psychol 1999;46:342–352.
45. Miller M. A bilinear multidimensional measurement model of Asian American acculturation and enculturation: Implications for counseling interventions. J Couns Psychol 2007;54:118–131.
46. Sodowsky G, Kwan K, Pannu R. Ethnic identity of Asians in the United States. In Ponterotto J. Casas J, Suzuki L, Alexander C. eds. *Handbook of Multicultural Counseling*. Thousand Oaks, CA: Sage, 1995:1123–1154.
47. Szapocznik J, Scopetta N, Kurtines W, Arandale M. Theory and measurement of acculturation. Interam J Psychol 1978;12:113–120.
48. Shim Y. The relationship between acculturation, cultural values, and cultural adjustment problems of Korean Americans. Diss Abstr 2005 l: Section B: The Sciences and Engineering. 65 (7-B):3774. U.S. University Microfilms International.
49. Choo B. Intergenerational conflict, family functioning, and acculturation experienced by Asian American community college students. Diss Abstr 2004 Section A: Humanit Soc Sci. 64 (12-A):4354.
50. Suinn R. SL-ASIA: Suinn-Lew Asian Self-Identity Acculturation Scale. Available at http://www.awong.com/~randy/dad/slasia.html 1994.

51. Park Y, Kim B. Asian and European cultural values and communication styles among Asian American and European American college students. Cultur Divers Ethnic Minor Psychol, 2008;14:47–56.
52. Kim B, Li L, Ng G. The Asian American Values Scale-Multidimensional: Development, reliability, and validity. Cultur Divers Ethnic Minor Psychol. 2005;11:187–201.
53. Chung R, Kim B, Abreu, J. Asian American Multidimensional Acculturation Scale: Development, factor analysis, reliability and validity. Cultur Divers Ethnic Minor Psychol 2004;10:66–80.
54. Yoo H, Lee R. Does ethnic identity buffer or exacerbate the effects of frequent racial discrimination on situational well-being of Asian-Americans? J Couns Psychol 2008;55:63–74.
55. Chen X, Unger J, Cruz T, Johnson C. Smoking patterns of Asian-American youth in California and their relationship with acculturation. J Adolesc Health 1999;24:321–328.
56. Herskovitz M. *Man and His Works: The Science of Cultural Anthropology*. NY: Knopf, 1948.
57. Kim B, Abreu J. Acculturation measurement: Theory, current instruments, and future directions. In Ponterotto J, Casas J, Suzuki L, Alexander C. eds. *Handbook of Multicultural Counseling*, 2nd ed. Thousand Oaks, CA: Sage, 2001:394–424.
58. Abe-Kim J, Okazaki S, Goto S. Unidimensional versus multidimensional approaches to the assessment of acculturation for Asian American populations. Cultur Divers Ethnic Minor Psychol 2001;7:232–246.
59. Mallinckrodt B, Shigeoka S, Suzuki L. Asian and Pacific Island American students' acculturation and etiology beliefs about typical counseling presenting problems. Cultur Divers Ethnic Minor Psychol 2005;11:227–238.
60. Kim S, Gonzales N, Stroh , Wang J. Parent–child cultural marginalization and depressive symptoms in Asian American family members. J Community Psychol 2006;34:167–182
61. LaFromboise T, Coleman H, Gerton J. Psychological impact of biculturalism: Evidence and theory. Psychol Bull 1993;114:395–412.
62. Nguyen, HH, Messe, LA, Stollak, GE. Toward a more complex understanding of acculturation and adjustment: Cultural involvements and psychosocial functioning in Vietnamese youth. J Cross Cult Psychol 1999; 30(1): 5–31.
63. Chun K, Morera O, Andal J, Skewes M. Conducting research with diverse Asian American groups. In Leong F, Inman F, Ebreo A, Yang L, Kinoshita L, Fu M. eds. *Handbook of Asian-American Psychology*. 2nd. ed. Thousand Oaks, CA: Sage, 2006:47–65.
64. Liao H, Rounds J, Klein A. A Test of Cramer's (1999) Help-seeking model and acculturation effects with Asian and Asian American college students. J Couns Psychol 2005;52:400–411.
65. Lau A, Jernewall N, Zane N, Myers H. Correlates of suicidal behaviors among Asian American outpatient youths. Cultur Divers Ethnic Minor Psychol 2002;8:199–213.
66. Wang C, Mallinckrodt B. Acculturation, attachment, and psychosocial adjustment of Chinese/Taiwanese International students. Cultur Divers Ethnic Minor Psychol 2006;53: 422–433.
67. Castelino P. Factors influencing career choices of South Asian Americans: A path analysis. Diss Abstr 2005. Section A: Humanities and Social Sciences. 65 (8-A):2906.
68. Hahm H, Lahiff M, Guterman N. Asian American adolescents' acculturation, binge drinking, and alcohol- and tobacco-using peers. J Community Psychol 2004;32:295–308.
69. Hahm H, Lahiff M, Guterman N. Acculturation and parental attachment in Asian-American adolescents' alcohol use. J Adolesc Health 2003;33:119–129.
70. Le T, Stockdale G. Acculturative dissonance, ethnic identity, and youth violence. Cultur Divers Ethnic Minor Psychol 2008;14:1–9.

Part II
Clinical Insights on Acculturation in Asian American Mental Health

The Impact of Immigration and Acculturation on the Mental Health of Asian Americans: Overview of Epidemiology and Clinical Implications

Siyon Rhee

Abstract In this chapter, we focus on an overview of clinical issues in Asian American mental health. In particular, we focus on psychological distress and its manifestation within different subpopulations, looking at common acculturation stressors as a background for understanding Asian American emotional health, as well as other key factors that are likely to affect Asian American mental health. We will review research on various age groups and clinical implications from the literature review, and finally, we look at what is known about mental health problems and mental health service utilization in Asian Americans.

Keywords Asian American mental health · Acculturation · Asian American mental health service utilization

Contents

Within-Group Diversity	82
Acculturation Stress Pertaining to Asian American Mental Health	83
Key Factors Affecting Asian American Mental Health	85
Language Barrier among Parents	85
Intergenerational Conflict	85
Identity Crisis	86
Domestic Violence	86
Prejudice and Discrimination	87
Epidemiology of Mental Health Problems among Asian Americans	87
Findings on Asian American Children and Youth	87
Findings on Immigrant Asian Adults	89
Findings on Immigrant Asian Older Adults	91
Use of Mental Health Services	93
Conclusion	94
References	94

S. Rhee (✉)
School of Social Work, California State University, Los Angeles, CA, USA
e-mail: srhee@calstatela.edu

Culture, historical events, environmental circumstances as well as migration-associated stressors can shape the mental health profile of any immigrant [1]. For example, the expression and recognition of psychiatric problems are fundamentally shaped by specific cultural practices. As mental illness is extremely stigmatizing in almost all Asian cultures, Asians are more likely to express somatic symptoms than Caucasian Americans in the presence of emotional or mental difficulties [2, 3]. For instance, Hwa-Byung (HB) or "suppressed anger syndrome," the literal translation of HB, is a widely held culture-bound folk syndrome among undereducated elderly immigrant Korean women who endure feelings of victimization within their oppressive patriarchal family structure and experience suppressed anger for an extensive period of time. Many of those experiencing HB report a variety of somatic as well as psychological symptoms including indigestion, headache, heat sensation, pressure sensations in the chest, epigastric mass, diminished concentration, and anxiety [4, 5]. In another example, over 90% of Cambodian refugees in the United States who experienced persecution and traumatic events during the 4 years of Pol Pot's regime (1975–1979) before coming to America were found to have developed posttraumatic stress disorder (PTSD).

It is difficult to establish the scope of psychiatric disorders among the Asian American population because of many obstacles, including cultural variations in the expression of mental health problems, the tremendous diversity and many internal differences within the population, and the lack of access to mental health services [1]. Although mental health researchers have begun to pay more attention to critical mental health issues facing this rapidly growing population, very little is known today about their precise need for mental health care, accessibility to mental health services, and the appropriateness of existing mental health services. Furthermore, most mental health studies tend to lump Asian Americans together as a homogeneous ethnic category. Thus, the amount of research and published materials on subgroup differences is particularly limited. Regardless, what follows will be a discussion of what is known and how this may impact the clinical care of these populations.

Within-Group Diversity

Asian Americans are extremely heterogeneous in terms of national origin, immigration status, educational level, economic status, generation, length of residence in the United States, and English proficiency along with cultural norms and values. For example, according to the most recent US Census statistics, Asians alone consisted of over 25 different ethnic groups [6]. Some Asian groups have predominantly middle-class backgrounds with high levels of educational attainment, whereas some other Asian groups, especially recent Indochinese refugees, are far less educated and much less able to speak English. Their literacy and transferable job skills are significantly lower than their Asian counterparts. Furthermore, although the annual median income of Asian American families is relatively high, there are a significant number of Asian American families who experience economic hardships and difficulties as they struggle with day-to-day survival in their new environments. Although race-based census data provide useful information about the overall picture of the group, they tend to ignore the within-group diversity. Nishioka [7] puts

> The Asian American community is highly diverse population, arguably more so than any other racial group. While some families have been in the United States for five generations or longer, many more are recent immigrants. From the Indian high-tech worker to the village farmer from Laos, they come to this country with varying degrees of education, skills, and financial resources (p. 34).

There are significant differences among ethnic Asian American groups in income and poverty rates. For example, there are significant differences in the amount of median family income between the more established groups and recent Southeast refugee groups. Similarly, the poverty rates from one group to another within the Asian American community vary widely. Specifically, in 1990, 14% of Chinese, 6.4% of Filipinos, 9.7% of Asian Indians, and 13.7% of Koreans lived below the poverty line, whereas the poverty rates for Vietnamese, Cambodians, and Hmong were consistently much higher than other Asian American groups, 25.7, 47.0, and 67.1%, respectively [8]. Furthermore, more than a quarter of Tongans, Samoans, and Bangladeshis live below the poverty line in Los Angeles County [9].

It is, therefore, difficult to generalize the life experiences and mental health issues of diverse Asian American groups, because they all have different social, cultural, and linguistic backgrounds, and also because their experiences and expectations change differentially as the length of residency in the United States increases. However, it has been generally assumed that cultural norms and values as well as socioeconomic backgrounds immigrants bring with them from their home countries have a significant impact on their psychological well-being in the process of adjusting to the new environment. For example, a 40-year-old recent immigrant from the Great Britain, compared with a recent immigrant of the same age from Cambodia, may be more easily acculturated and accepted into the dominant European American mainstream linguistically, socially, and culturally. Uba and Sue conclude, "such diversity suggests that different groups have varying needs for social services and that services would be most effectively provided in ways that are tailored for each group" [10].

Acculturation Stress Pertaining to Asian American Mental Health

According to Hurh and Kim's [11] four phases of adaptation, most new Asian immigrants initially experience constraints or *exigency*, the first phase of adaptation, during the first couple of years of relocation. This stage is characterized by the challenges of language barriers, unemployment or underemployment, social isolation, and culture shock. The second phase is *resolution* stage (2 to 10–15 years) during which the immigrants' life satisfaction may reach its peak. The third phase is *social marginality* characterized by the stagnation in life satisfaction due to identity crisis stemming from feelings of relative deprivation and marginality from the mainstream. The last phase of adaptation is *marginality acceptance*, or finally, development of a *new identity*.

Immigration to a new country undoubtedly can be a stressful life experience that can lead to "cultural shock" [12], "migration stress," [13] and "acculturative stress" [14, 15]. These types of stress have various mental health consequences, including affective disorders, anxiety, and adjustment difficulties. Although the majority of Asian immigrants and refugees stay emotionally healthy, a significant proportion of this population develops mental health problems. The most frequently diagnosed mental disorders in this population are depression, PTSD, anxiety disorders, and schizophrenia.

Asian Americans have been portrayed as the "model minority" by the media for more than three decades because of their relatively high educational, occupational, and economic attainments and low criminal activity and dependence on public welfare. This national conception has created images of Asian Americans as a well-adjusted and adapted minority group among the general public as well as mental health professionals [16–18]. Such a stereotypical view has important consequences in mental health service delivery and research. For example, it has been generally assumed that Asians have few mental health problems, and that they have resources within the family or ethnic community to meet their mental health needs. This popular belief has served to justify the lack of attention to their unique psychological needs. Consequently, the amount of research conducted with Asian American national samples focusing on the prevalence of mental disorders and patterns of service utilization is extremely limited, compared with other ethnic minority groups.

It is well known that immigrant Asian families can exhibit a broad range of strengths such as high educational achievements, above-average median income, emphasis on family cohesiveness and support, occupational upward mobility, and emphasis on the value of hard work. At the same time, this population is also exposed to a number of vulnerable mental health risk factors. Emotional well-being and mental health are affected not only by organic factors but also by a number of psychosocial stressors and a lack of adequate resources. It is generally assumed that levels of acculturation usually measured by the length of residency in the United States and the ability to speak English can moderate the negative impact of pre-migration traumatic experiences (PTE) on the psychological well-being among immigrants. Ngo et al. [19] conducted a study with a community-based sample of 261 adult Vietnamese Americans and found that PTE had a strong effect on depression among those with lower levels of acculturation than those who were highly acculturated. Thus, PTE tends to induce higher levels of depressive symptoms, whereas its effect is weaker among those refugees who have been in the United States for a longer period of time.

Key Factors Affecting Asian American Mental Health

Most Asian immigrants, especially during the early stage of relocation, experience a variety of difficulties stemming from the difference in language, migratory grief, social isolation, unfamiliarity with Western customs, values and laws, limited social support, declined social status, and inability to participate in mainstream social and political activities. These difficulties are experienced by the majority of Asian immigrants regardless of their age and socioeconomic background [10, 20]. Some of the most common stressors facing immigrant Asian children, adults, and elders that have some bearing on Asian American mental health are as follows:

Language Barrier among Parents

For many Asian immigrants, English remains as an almost impossible language to master because of the vast linguistic differences between the two languages. Lack of work experience in America and insufficient English skills make white-collar occupations far less accessible to Asian immigrants despite their advanced educational backgrounds. This explains why Asian immigrants turn to highly competitive family-run small businesses that require a husband and a wife to work more than 12 h a day, 7 days a week. A critical issue facing many Asian American immigrants, especially the male heads of households, is the high level of stress and low self-esteem resulting from status inconsistency and extended work hours without having vacations for many years. Apparently, communication difficulties due to the differences in English proficiency and cultural values between parents and children have become a common feature among many immigrant Asian American families throughout the nation [21]. A recent study suggests that immigrant parents' language proficiency correlates significantly with indicators of intergenerational conflict and adolescent psychological well-being in immigrant Chinese American families, that is, the less proficient their English, the more conflict arises [22].

Intergenerational Conflict

Asian culture places great value on hierarchical order, respect for seniors, family obligations, filial piety, and obedience to rules and authority [23]. Immigrant Asian families tend to be highly male-dominant and define females and children as subordinate to their male head of the household. Children are expected to show unquestioning obedience to their parents' needs and wishes. The traditional values held by the Asian immigrants at the time of arrival are likely to be modified as they interact with people in the American mainstream. However, the fundamental belief system tends to remain relatively unchanged. It has been well documented in the research literature that there exists a wide range of cultural gaps between the foreign-born parents, who are likely to adhere to their traditional values, and their US-born or US-raised adolescents, who are exposed to conflicting mainstream values [24–26].

Overshadowed by the popular positive image of Asian American students and high levels of academic achievement among a portion of this group, their problem behaviors have often been overlooked in educational as well as research communities. Emotional difficulties are particularly pressing issues for many Asian American adolescents who face the challenge of successful psychosocial adjustment to the host society, and, simultaneously, who are expected to value and maintain their heritage through socialization with immigrant parents and members of their ethnic community [25].

Identity Crisis

Ethnic identity development is particularly critical for minority adolescents as they have, in addition to their ordinary developmental issues, an added burden of exploring the values of both host society and their original cultures and integrating them into their own identities. There is a significant relationship between positive attitudes toward one's own ethnic group and the positive psychological well-being among ethnic minority adolescents. More specifically, maintaining a positive identification with both one's own and the host society's culture predicts higher levels of positive psychological outcomes for adolescents [27, 28]. As mentioned previously, Asian American children are expected to value and maintain their heritage through socialization with immigrant parents and members of their ethnic community and, at the same time, to learn quickly the language and certain behavioral patterns of the host society in the adaptation process. For instance, immigrant Asian parents emphasize obedience and conformity with parental expectations and yet, paradoxically, may recognize the importance of individual autonomy and self-assertion for the academic and social success of their children in the host society [25, 26, 29]. In this process, Asian American children often experience a serious problem of identity crisis and frustration between the two cultures, which may be related to a variety of emotional and behavioral difficulties.

Domestic Violence

Contrary to their general stereotype of a model minority, immigrant Asian American families are reported to experience high rates of spousal abuse among various ethnic groups throughout the nation [30–32]. For example, the Korean Family Service Center [33] in Los Angeles reported that domestic violence was one of the leading reasons to seek help from the agency among immigrant Korean families. In Hawaii, Samoan adults and Native Hawaiian men were overrepresented as perpetrators of child maltreatment and spouse abuse, respectively, in proportion to the total population size [30]. A recent study shows a high level of verbal aggression perpetrated by Chinese men toward their spouse or intimate partners, implying that certain Asian men do not necessarily view marital violence as a violation of a woman's rights [34]. Another study, which examined wife abuse attitudes among immigrant Cambodian, Chinese, Korean, and Vietnamese adults living in the United States, demonstrates that as high as 24–36% of the sample agreed that violence is justified in certain situations such as a wife's sexual infidelity, her nagging, or her refusal to cook or clean [35].

Prejudice and Discrimination

Goto et al. [36] report that one in five Chinese Americans experiences discrimination based on race, ethnicity, language, or accent; as high as 43% of these types of incidents occurred within the past year. In addition, Asian Americans face a variety of issues of social and institutional racism that are unique to them. For example, owing to their physical appearance, lifestyles, and values, Asians are frequently perceived as "perpetual foreigners" [36, 37]. US-born Asians are often being told they "speak English so well," and they are frequently asked where they are *really* from (when answering "Where is your family from?" with "Los Angeles," they are asked again "No, where is your family really/originally from?").

Development of a positive self-concept and a secure sense of ethnic identity are influenced by the quality of interactions between individuals and their larger social environment [38, 39]. As members of ethnic minority groups, Asian American children and youths as well as adults are often confronted with a systemic issue of racial discrimination and unfair treatment, which may negatively influence their psychological and behavioral development. "Often, Asian Americans, no matter how long they have been in the United States, regardless of citizenship, have to deal with rampant cultural and institutional racism as well as individual racism (10 p. 6)." Particularly, Asian American adolescents' perception of their ethnic/racial status in larger society and awareness of prejudice and discrimination against their ethnic groups are likely to undermine their ethnic pride, which may contribute to their psychological distress and further contribute to feelings of social isolation, inferiority, and inadequacy [28, 29, 40].

Epidemiology of Mental Health Problems among Asian Americans

Findings on Asian American Children and Youth

Asian American children and adolescents with immigrant backgrounds often report feelings of confusion, anger, and frustration attributable to relationship difficulties with their traditional parents [24, 41]. In the 1980s, Sue and Morishma [42] found that Asian American students exhibited higher levels of anxiety than non-Asian students. Studies have reported an increasing rate of depression, school dropout, substance abuse, and juvenile delinquency among Asian American adolescents [17, 43–47].

Recently, Ying and Han [48] examined the intergenerational gap in acculturation, subsequent conflicts, and their mental health consequences among 490 Southeast Asian American adolescents using data from the Children of Immigrants Longitudinal Study. The primary hypothesis of their research was that perceived intergenerational gap and discrepancy in acculturation in early adolescence among Asian American adolescents would predict intergenerational conflict in late adolescence, which, in turn, would increase the likelihood of developing depression in late adolescence. Initial survey data were collected from Southeast Asian American adolescents in 8th and 9th grades, and the same respondents completed the surveys again in 3 years. The results demonstrated that intergenerational conflict significantly mediated the effect of perceived acculturation gap on the development of depression symptoms among later-staged adolescents. The study suggests an importance of intervention/prevention programs for both parents and adolescents in the Asian community.

Various groups of Asian American students share common cultural backgrounds as well as the unique experience of discrimination and prejudice associated with being a minority in the United States. Asaman and Berry's study [49] of Japanese American and Chinese American college students found that Japanese American students who perceived more racial prejudice against them were more likely to have a lower self-esteem than those who perceived less racial prejudice. Shrake and Rhee [28] examined ethnic identity and perceived discrimination as predictors of adolescent problem behaviors among Korean American adolescents. According to their findings, level of ethnic identity, perceived discrimination, and academic performance are significant predictors of both internalizing and externalizing problems. Ethnic identity, in this study, was defined as a sense of belonging and positive attachment to one's ethnic group. Internalizing problems were operationally defined as exhibiting anxiety, depression, and somatic complaints, whereas externalizing problems included aggressive and delinquent behaviors. Their findings indicate [1] the higher their sense of belonging to their ethnic group, the lower the problem behaviors; [2] the prevalence of problem behaviors is highly associated with adolescents' perceptions of racial discrimination; and [3] adolescents who reported higher Grade Point Average (GPAs) tended to have fewer delinquency problems.

Perhaps, Asian American students who perpetrate delinquent acts and behave aggressively may have been subject to multiple accounts of discrimination as if they were inferior, second-class citizens. They may develop low self-esteem and a strong sense of anger and frustration toward their multiethnic environment at an early age. Ethnocultural interviews conducted with Asian American adolescents in probation by the author have revealed that they frequently mention unpleasant racially based experiences as a part of their problems.

Some researchers and practitioners have argued that the highly competitive journey toward academic excellence can adversely contribute to significant psychological distress for some Asian American adolescents as a result of the tremendous amount of stress and pressure from their families and teachers [50]. Despite the popular belief that Asian American students' high academic achievement comes with heavy psychological costs, many studies affirm that involvement in academic activities promotes psychosocial adjustment and is likely to prevent a variety of maladaptive and deviant behaviors [51, 52]. These studies demonstrate evidence that high academic performance enhances adolescents' self-esteem and personal efficacy by providing them with more adaptive means of handling personal or contextual challenges and obstacles. For example, according to Chen and Stevenson's study [51] conducted with a large sample of cross-cultural subjects, there was no evidence that highly achieving Asian American students experienced a greater frequency of maladjustment symptoms than European American counterparts.

Aldwin and Greenberger [53] conducted a comparative study on the level of depression among Korean and European American college students. According to their findings, Korean students were significantly more depressed than their European American counterparts, and the respondents' perceived parental traditionalism was related to higher levels of depression among the Korean sample. Recently, Okazaki [54] measured differences in depression and social anxiety among Asian American (mostly Chinese, Korean, and Japanese) and European American college students (N = 348; 165 Asian Americans and 183 European Americans). She found in this study that Asian students scored significantly higher than European American students on both measures of depression and anxiety. Abe and Zane [55] examined cross-cultural differences between European American and foreign-born Asian American college students on a measure of psychological maladjustment. Results from this study show that foreign-born Asian respondents had higher levels of interpersonal distress than their European American counterparts. These studies provide evidence that Asian American youth have comparable, if not higher, rates of difficulties in mental health.

Findings on Immigrant Asian Adults

It is important to note at this juncture that mental health problems can be measured by symptom scales rather than by standardized DSM criteria, which rely strictly both on the presence of symptoms and on the intensity and duration of the symptoms for more accurate diagnosis [1]. In current research, much is known about Asian American mental health problems of adults and older adults as measured by symptom scales than by those measured to generate DSM diagnostic categories.

In studies utilizing depressive symptom scales, respondents are often asked to report whether or not they have indicators of depressive symptoms (yes/no) and how many days they experienced them in the past week. For example, Kuo's study [45], which utilized symptom measures and not DSM criteria, reveals that a community sample of Chinese-, Filipino-, Japanese-, and Korean-Americans recruited from various community settings in Seattle exhibited slightly more depressive symptoms than did European Americans.

Kuo and Tsai [56] report several other important findings on the psychological well-being of Asian immigrants. In their study, it was found that there were significant interethnic differences in the level of depression among various immigrant Asian groups. The Koreans, the most recently arrived immigrants, were found to exhibit depressive symptoms significantly more than the Chinese-, Filipino-, and Japanese-Americans. For the overall sample, immigrants who came to the United States at a younger age had fewer adjustment difficulties. Asian immigrants with "hardy" personalities or those who maintain a sense of control over their life activities tend to perceive immigration as an opportunity for personal development and adjust more adaptively to their new environment. In addition, Asian immigrants who report to have a stable network of social support, including relatives and friends living close to their residence, display fewer depressive symptoms than did those who do not have such resources. Findings from Hurh and Kim's research [57] are consistent with those from Kuo and Tsai's study. In their study, Korean immigrants in Chicago scored significantly higher on depression measures than did the Chinese, Filipinos, and Japanese. Ying's study [58], conducted with a sample drawn from various community organizations in San Francisco using the Center for Epidemiologic Studies – Depression Scale (CES-D Scale), suggests that Chinese immigrants, especially from a lower socioeconomic background, were significantly more depressed than the European Americans and the Chinese Americans in Kuo's study.

It has been well documented that Southeast Asian refugees constitute a high-risk group for a broad range of mental disorders [59–61]. The impact of traumatic life-threatening events tends to be extensive and lifelong among refugees, regardless of the length of stay in this country. Blair [60] points out that the frequency and intensity of traumas experienced by refugees affect the rate of PTSD in the refugee population. Blair examined the mental health status and risk factors associated with a diagnosis of PTSD among a random sample of 124 Cambodian refugee adults. The most notable findings include that experiencing a greater number of war traumas, such as loss of immediate family members, and experiencing a greater number of resettlement stressors increased the risk of PTSD in the Cambodian refugee population.

Considerable evidence from mental health studies using various symptom scales suggests that immigrant Asians or Asian Americans experience significantly high levels of distress, consistent with depression, PTSD, anxiety, and somatoform disorder [3, 62–64]. Two major large-scale mental health studies, the Epidemiological Catchment Area (ECA) study and the National Comorbidity Study (NCS), examined the prevalence of lifetime DSM-III or DSM-IIIR psychiatric disorders in the US population in the 1980s using the Diagnostic Interview Schedule (DIS). It was found that there was a relatively low prevalence of most psychiatric disorders among Asian Americans as compared with European American adults. However, these studies only selected English-speaking Asians as a single ethnic category, and Asians comprised less than a significant proportion of the total sample. Therefore, it appears that the results from these studies are not adequate for Asian population estimates and are not representative of the diverse picture of immigrant Asian and Asian American mental health needs. In addition, these studies used scales that were diagnoses-based and not symptom-based.

The Chinese American Psychiatric Epidemiological Study (CAPES) was the first methodologically rigorous large-scale research study designed to estimate the prevalence of selected psychiatric disorders using DSM-IIIR criteria among immigrant Chinese Americans predominantly. Similar to the ECA study that used one geographic site instead of a national sample, CAPES was implemented in the Los Angeles area and 1,747 face-to-face interviews in various Chinese dialects were conducted in 1993–1994. Like the ECA and NCS studies, this study used the University of Michigan Version of the Composite International Diagnostic Interview Schedule (UM-CIDI) to yield major DSM diagnoses in the immigrant Chinese population. According to Takeuchi and colleagues [65], 6.9% of the Chinese respondents had major depression during their lifetime as compared with the 17.1% lifetime prevalence rate for Americans found in the NCS study [66] and 4.9% among Americans in the ECA study [67]. A consistent pattern for dysthymic disorder was also found in the Chinese population. About 5% of the Chinese respondents reported to have dysthymia during their lifetime, whereas 6.4% of the American respondents in the NCS study and 3.2% in the ECA study reported to have such a diagnosis. However, interestingly, the lifetime rates of anxiety disorders, phobia, and panic disorder were generally lower than those found in the other two major surveys.

More recently, Takeuchi and colleagues [68] conducted the National Latino and Asian American Study, the first national epidemiological survey of Asian Americans in the United States. In this national sample of Asian Americans, they examined the lifetime and 12-month prevalence rates of depressive, anxiety, and substance abuse disorders using the World Health Organization Composite International DIS. One of their significant findings includes that immigration-related factors, such as nativity (US-born versus foreign-born), have some influence on mental disorders for Asian Americans. However, the relationships between these two dimensions were different for men and women. More acculturated Asian men with the ability to speak English fluently were found to have lower rates of lifetime and 12-month disorders compared with non-English-speaking men. On the other hand, interestingly, immigrant women had lower rates of any of those mental disorders as compared with US-born Asian American women. It was speculated that fluent English speakers may have more affluent socioeconomic backgrounds than those who do not speak the language well.

Findings on Immigrant Asian Older Adults

Depression has been reported to be the most prevalent affective disorder found in the elderly population across almost all ethnic groups in the United States

[69, 70]. Immigrants, particularly those with no close kinship ties and social support network due to relocation, are more likely to experience life stresses and increased mental health risks than US-born Americans. Studies have shown that elderly Asian immigrants are at a higher risk of developing depression than their non-Hispanic European American counterparts [58, 71–74]. More specifically, the mean scores of depressive symptoms among immigrant Asian elders have been found to be generally higher than non-Asian older adults or at least similar to those found in other community samples of older people.

Results from one of Mui's studies [73] on depression among Korean elderly using the Brink et al. cutoff points of the Geriatric Depression Scale (GDS) show that 35.8% of immigrant Korean elderly in her study were mildly depressed, whereas 9% were moderately-to-severely depressed. Mui's other study [72] looking at depression among immigrant Chinese elderly in New York reveals that 18% of the respondents were mildly-to-severely depressed. Mui [72, 73] also found that elderly Chinese and Korean immigrants who rated their health as good, who lived with someone, and who were satisfied with help received from family members were less likely to be depressed than those who reported differently on these items. Consistently, another recent study on screening for depression in immigrant Chinese American elders shows that health status, poverty, length of residence, educational attainment, and English ability were significant predictors of depression for this population [75]. This study suggests that good health, middle-to-high income, long-term residence, advanced education, and proficient English ability have something to do with lower levels of depression in this population. Casado and Leung [20] also found that migratory grief and loss, poor language proficiency, and the higher degree of attachment to one's home country significantly affect the development of depressive symptoms among elderly Chinese immigrants.

Wu et al. [76] assessed the effects of various chronic illnesses on depression in a community sample of immigrant Chinese elders. Results from their study show that, although women report slightly higher depression scores than men, the difference in the overall depression scores between the two groups is not statistically significant. Gender is not a predictor for depressive symptoms in the multivariate models. It is possible that the immigration process for many elderly Chinese males may have weakened their authority within the family or may have even reversed their status as the head of the household. Consequently, elderly Chinese immigrant men may have experienced higher levels of depressive symptoms than US-born Chinese counterparts or those in their homeland.

The above studies, which used symptom scales and not DSM criteria-based scales, show higher levels of depressive symptoms among immigrant Asian elderly as compared with European American older adults. Yamamoto et al. [77] conducted an ECA type of survey with a small sample of 100 immigrant Korean elderly to examine the lifetime prevalence of various DSM-III mental disorders. Unlike the above studies, this study found a relatively low prevalence of lifetime mental disorders in this population with an exception of alcohol abuse and dependence. The lifetime prevalence of major depression among immigrant Korean elders was found to be 1.0%, and the lifetime prevalence of dysthymic disorder was 2.0%.

Depression is one of the most significant risk factors associated with suicide in late life [1, 78]. Asian elderly immigrants are generally at a much higher risk of suicide than US-born Asian older adults. Yu [79] reported that the suicide rate for elderly Chinese immigrants was almost three times higher than that for US-born Chinese elderly in 1980. It is highly probable that depression occurs more frequently among elderly immigrants because they tend to experience a wider range of adjustment difficulties, including inability to speak English, limited access to resources, stressful life events, separation from significant others, loss of status, and social isolation. In recent years, the number of suicide cases among immigrant Korean elderly had significantly increased in the Los Angeles area where the highest concentration of Korean immigrants in the United States is found.

Use of Mental Health Services

As previously suggested, mental health problems among the Asian American population have been generally underestimated across various Asian ethnic groups. Considerable evidence suggests that mental disorders and emotional disturbances among Asian Americans are at least as prevalent as those among non-Hispanic European Americans [10, 16]. Furthermore, a number of research findings indicate that certain categories of mental disturbance, such as PTSD and adjustment disorder, are much more prevalent among particular Asian groups including Cambodians, Vietnamese, and Hmong refugees.

Despite the evidence of high rates of mental health problems among the immigrant Asian populations, Asians are far less likely to utilize mental health services, as compared with other ethnic/racial group members [42, 80–83]. Matsuoka et al. [84], in their examination of national formal service utilization rates, demonstrate that Asian Americans were three times less likely to utilize mental health services than their European American counterparts. In addition, those who manage to come to the attention of mental health professionals tend to exhibit more severe and chronic symptoms in comparison with non-Asians [85, 86]. Thus, evidence indicates that Asian Americans, when they use formal mental health care, tend to initiate treatment much later and terminate treatment more prematurely than non-Hispanic European Americans. A variety of reasons, cultural or systemic, contribute to this delayed initiation of treatment process, such as loss of face and stigma attached to admission of mental illness, lack of bicultural/bilingual mental health professionals, and incompatibility of widely practiced Western mental health treatment models.

Conclusion

Of the 12.5 million Asian Americans today, more than two-thirds are foreign-born residents. As such, it is helpful to bear in mind that those Asians with immigrant backgrounds are extremely diverse, particularly in terms of socio-economic status, generation, and length of residence. The life experiences and mental health issues brought by Asian American clients will vary widely from one group to another. Therefore, any stereotypical conceptions held by mental health practitioners that Asians comprise one homogeneous ethnic category may lead to erroneous diagnoses as well as to ineffective intervention strategies. The variations in their backgrounds are likely to contribute to differential symptom manifestation and expression, which will require the mental health professionals' sensitivity and keen insight.

In addition, new immigrants usually go through a few exclusive phases of adaptation. Each stage of adaptation represents different life challenges (e.g., newcomers may struggle with linguistic difficulties, isolation and loneliness, whereas more-acculturated individuals are more likely to experience issues stemming from identity crises). Therefore, in providing services to Asian American clients, mental health professionals need to consider a client's stage of acculturation as a vital factor in selecting phase-appropriate intervention approaches.

Numerous studies reveal that racial disparities exist in mental health service utilization. It has been generally indicated that the prevalence of mental disorders among Asian Americans is at least as high as that of non-Hispanic European Americans. Nonetheless, utilization of formal mental health services among Asian Americans is significantly lower as compared with non-Asian groups. There are numerous factors and barriers that have been previously suggested that influence help-seeking behaviors and attitudes, such as cultural barriers (shame for seeking help, stigma, loss of face, distrust toward Western treatment models, etc.) and practical/structural barriers (cost, inaccessibility due to lack of transportation, lack of awareness of services, etc.). According to a recent study, the majority of an immigrant Asian group surveyed indicated the structural/practical barriers (cost, language incompatibility, transportation, and lack of knowledge of available services) as the major obstacles to seeking treatment [87]. Although we need to be cautious in generalizing such findings, there is convincing evidence that future collaborations amongst researchers, mental health clinicians, and policy makers will move us closer to providing the kind of services necessary for the successful treatment of Asian Americans.

References

1. Office of the Surgeon General. Mental health: Culture, race, ethnicity – supplement. U.S. Department of Health and Human Services, SAMHSA 1999. Retrieved October 30, 2006 from http://www.mentalhealth.samhsa.gov/cre/default.asp
2. Hsu LKG, Folstein MF. Somatoform disorders in Caucasian and Chinese Americans. The Journal of Nervous and Mental Disease 1997; 185: 382–387.

3. Kleinman A. Depression, somatization and the new cross-cultural psychiatry. Social Science & Medicine 1977; 11: 3–10.
4. Lin KM, Lau JKC, Yamamoto J, Zheng Y, Kim H, Cho K, Nakasaki G. Hwa-Byung: A community study of Korean Americans. The Journal of Nervous and Mental Disorder 1992; 180: 386–391.
5. Park Y, Kim HS, Schwartz-Barcott D, Kim J. The conceptual structure of Hwa-Byung in middle-aged Korean women. Health Care for Women International 2002; 23: 389–398.
6. U.S. Census Bureau (2002). *The Asian population 2000: Census 2000 brief.* Retrieved October 24, 2005 from http://www.census.gov/prod/2002pubs/c2kbr01-16.pdf
7. Nishioka J. Socioeconomics: The model minority? In: Lai E, Arguelles D, eds. The New Face of Asian Pacific America: Numbers, Diversity & Change in the 21st Century. Los Angeles, CA: UCLA Asian American Studies Center Press, 2003: 29–35.
8. Lai E, Arguelles D. The New Face of Asian Pacific America: Numbers, Diversity & Change in the 21st Century, Los Angeles, CA: UCLA Asian American Studies Center Press, 2003.
9. Asian Pacific American Legal Center of Southern California. The Diverse Face of Asians and Pacific Islanders in Los Angeles County, 2004. Retrieved on 12 July 2004 from http://www.unitedwayla.org/pages/rpts_resource/ethnic_profiles/ASP_Report.pdf
10. Uba L, Sue S. Nature and scope of services for Asian and Pacific Islander Americans. In: Mokuau N, ed. Handbook of Social Services for Asian and Pacific Islanders. Westport, CT: Green Press, 1991: 3–19.
11. Hurh WM, Kim KC. Adaptation stages and mental health of Korean male immigrants in the United States. International Migration Review 1990; 24: 456–479.
12. Oberg K. Culture shock: Adjustment to new cultural environments. Practical Anthropology 1960; 7: 177–182.
13. Beiser M. Migration in a developing country: Risk and opportunity. In: R. C. Nann, ed. Uprooting and Surviving: Adaptation and Resettlement of Migrant Families and Children. Dordrecht: Reidel, 1982: 119–146.
14. Berry JW. Acculturation and psychological adaptation. In: Kim YY, Gudtkunst WB, eds. Current Studies in Cross-Cultural Adaptation. London: Sage, 1987: 29–44.
15. Berry JW, Sam D. Acculturation and adaptation. In: Berry JW, ed. Handbook of Cross-Cultural Psychology, Vol. 3. Boston, MA: Allyn & Bacon, 1997: 291–316.
16. Lee J, Lei A, Sue S. The current state of mental health research on Asian Americans. Journal of Human Behavior in the Social Environment 2001; 3: 159–178.
17. Lee CL, Zane NWS. An overview. In: Lee CL & Zane NWS, ed. Handbook of Asian American Psychology. Thousand Oaks, CA: Sage, 1998: 1–19.
18. Sue S, Sue DW, Sue L, Takeuchi DT. Psychopathology among Asian Americans: A model minority? Cultural Diversity and Mental Health 1995; 1: 39–54.
19. Ngo D, Tran TV, Gibbons JL, Oliver JM. Acculturation, premigration traumatic experiences, and depression among Vietnamese Americans. Journal of Human Behavior in the Social Environment 2001; 3: 225–242.
20. Casado B, Leung P. Migratory grief and depression among elderly Chinese American immigrants. Journal of Gerontological Social Work 2001; 36: 5–26.
21. Rhee S, Chang J, Rhee J. Acculturation, communication patterns, and self-esteem among Asian and Caucasian American adolescents. Adolescence 2003; 38: 749–768.
22. Lim SL. Acculturation Consonance and Dissonance: Effect on Parenting Style, Parent-Adolescent Relationship, and Adolescent Psychological Well-Being in Immigrant Chinese-American Families. Doctoral dissertation submitted to Texas Tech University, USA. 2002.
23. Kitano HL, Daniels R. Asian Americans: Emerging minorities. Englewood Cliffs, NJ: Prentice Hall, 1995.
24. Lee E. Working with Asian Americans: A guide for clinicians. New York: Guilford Press, 1997.

25. Rhee S. Effective social work practice with Korean immigrant families. Journal of Multicultural Social Work 1996; 4: 49–61.
26. Ying YW. Strengthening intergenerational/intercultural ties in migrant families: A new intervention for parents. Journal of Community Psychology 1998; 27: 89–96.
27. Phinney JS, Chavira V, Williamson L. Acculturation attitudes and self-esteem among high school and college students. Youth & Society 1992; 23: 299–312.
28. Shrake EK & Rhee S. Ethnic identity as a predictor of problem behaviors among Korean American adolescents. Adolescence 2004; 39: 601–622.
29. Uba L. Asian Americans: Personality patterns, identity, and mental health. New York: Guilford Press, 1994.
30. Furuto SM. (1991). Family violence among Pacific Islanders. In: Mokuau N, ed. Handbook of Social Services for Asian and Pacific Islanders. Westport, CT: Green Press, 1991: 203–215.
31. Rhee S. Domestic violence in the Korean immigrant families. Journal of Sociology and Social Welfare 1997; 24: 63–77.
32. Sue D. Asian American/Pacific Islander families in conflict. In: Barrett KH, George WH, eds. Race, Culture, Psychology, and Law. Thousand Oaks, CA: Sage, 2005: 257–268.
33. Korean American Family Service Center. Annual statistics, 2004. Los Angeles, CA.
34 Yick AG, Shibusawa T, Agbayani-Siewert P. Partner violence, depression, and practice implications with families of Chinese descent. Journal of Cultural Diversity 2003; 10: 96–104.
35. Yoshioka MR, Dinoia J, Ullah K. Attitudes toward marital violence: An examination of four Asian communities. Violence Against Women 2001; 7: 900–927.
36. Goto SG, Gee GC, Takeuchi DT. Strangers still? The experience of discrimination among Chinese Americans. Journal of Community Psychology 2002; 30: 211–224.
37. Dhooper SS, Moore SE. Social Work Practice with Culturally Diverse People. Thousand Oaks, CA: Sage, 2001.
38. Pinderhughes E. Afro-American families and the victim system. In: McGoldrick M, Pearce JK, Giordana J, eds. Ethnicity and Family Therapy. New York: Guilford, 1982: 108–122.
39. Schaefer RT. Racial and Ethnic groups, 8th ed. Upper Saddle River, NJ: Prentice Hall, 2002.
40. Phinney JS, Kohatsu E. Ethnic and racial identity development and mental health. In: Schulenberg J, Maggs JL, Herrelmann K, eds. Health Risks and Developmental Transitions during Adolescence. Cambridge, MA: Cambridge University Press, 1997: 420–443.
41. Ho MK. Minority children and adolescents in therapy. Newbury Park, CA: Sage, 1992.
42. Sue S, Morishma JK. The mental health of Asian Americans. San Francisco, CA: Jossey-Bass, 1982.
43. Ja D, Yuen FK. Substance abuse treatment among Asian Americans. In: Lee E, ed. Working with Asian Americans. New York: Guilford Press, 1997: 295–308.
44. Kim TE, Goto SG. Peer delinquency and parental social support and predictors of Asian American adolescent delinquency. Deviant Behavior: An Interdisciplinary Journal 2000; 21: 331–347.
45. Kuo WH. Prevalence of depression among Asian Americans. Journal of Nervous and Mental Disease 1984; 172: 449–457.
46. Lorenzo M, Pakiz B, Reinherz H, Frost A. Emotional and behavioral problems of Asian American adolescents: A comparative study. Child and Adolescent Social Work Journal 1995; 12: 195–212.
47. Tamaki J. Cultural balancing act adds to teen angst. Los Angeles Times, 13 July 1998.
48. Ying YW, Han MK. The longitudinal effect of intergenerational gap in acculturation on conflict and mental health in Southeast Asian American adolescents. American Journal of Orthopsychiatry 2007; 77: 61–66.
49. Asaman J, Berry G. Self-concept, alienation, and perceived prejudice: Implications for counseling Asian Americans. Journal of Multicultural Counseling and Development 1987; 15: 146–161.

50. Lee S. Behind the model-minority stereotype: Voices of high- and low-achieving Asian American students. Anthropology & Educational Quarterly 1994; 25: 413–429.
51. Chen C, Stevenson HW. Motivation and mathematics achievement: A comparative study of Asian-American, Caucasian-American, and East Asian high school students. Child Development 1995; 66: 1215–1234.
52. Sue S, Okazaki S. Asian-American educational achievements: A phenomenon in search of an explanation. American Psychologist 1990; 45: 913–920.
53. Aldwin C, Greenberger E. Cultural differences in the predictors of depression. American Journal of Community Psychology 1987; 15: 789–813.
54. Okazaki S. Sources of ethnic differences between Asian American and White American college students on measures of depression and social anxiety. Journal of Abnormal Psychology 1997; 106: 52–60.
55. Abe JS, Zane NW. Psychological maladjustment among Asian and White American college students: Controlling for confounds. Journal of Counseling Psychology 1990; 37: 437–444.
56. Kuo WH, Tsai YM. Social networking, hardiness, and immigrants' mental health. Journal of Health and Social Behavior 1986; 27: 133–149.
57. Hurh WM, Kim KC. Uprooting and adjustment: A sociological study of Korean immigrants' mental health. Final report to the National Institute of Mental Health. Macomb, IL: Department of Sociology and Anthropology, Western Illinois University, 1988.
58. Ying YW. Depressive symptomatology among Chinese-Americans as measured by the CES-D. Journal of Clinical Psychology 1988; 44: 739–746.
59. Bemak F, Chung RC, Bornemann T. Counseling and psychotherapy with refugees. In: Pedersen PB, Draguns JG, Walter WJ, Trimble JE, ed. Counseling across Cultures, 4th ed. Thousand Oaks, CA: Sage, 1996: 243–265.
60. Blair R. Risk factors associated with PTSD and major depression among Cambodian refugees in Utah. Health & Social Work 2000; 25: 23–30.
61. Kinzie JD, Leung PK, Boehnlein JK. Treatment of depressive disorders in refugees. In Lee E, ed. Working with Asian Americans: A guide for Clinicians. New York: The Guildford Press, 1997: 265–294.
62. Hsu LKG, Folstein, MF. Somatoform disorders in Caucasian and Chinese Americans. Journal of Nervous and Mental Disease 1997; 185: 382–387.
63. Iwamasa GY. Asian Americans. In: Friedman S, ed. Cultural Issues in the Treatment of Anxiety. New York: Guilford Press, 1997: 99–129.
64. Tran TV. Psychological traumas and depression in a sample of Vietnamese people in the United States. Health and Social Work 1993; 18: 184–194.
65. Takeuchi DT, Chung RC, Lin KM, Shen H, Kurasaki K, Chun CA, Sue S. Lifetime and twelve-month prevalence rates of major depressive episodes and dysthymia among Chinese Americans in Los Angeles. American Journal of Psychiatry 1998; 155: 1407–1414.
66. Kessler RC, McGonagle KA, Zhao S, Nelson CB, Hughes M, Eshleman S, Wittchen H, Kendler KS. Lifetime and 12-month prevalence of DSM-III-R psychiatric disorders in the United States. Archives of General Psychiatry 1994; 51: 8–19.
67. Robins LN, Regier DA. Psychiatric Disorders in America: The Epidemiological Catchment Area Study. New York: Free Press, 1991.
68. Takeuchi DT, Zane N, Hong S, Chae DH, Gong F, Gee GC, Walton E, Sue S, Alegria M. Immigration-related factors and mental disorders among Asian American. American J of Public Health 2007; 97: 84–90.
69. Blazer DG, Koening HG. Mood disorders. In: Busses EW, Blazer DG, ed. Textbook of Geriatric Psychiatry, 2nd ed. Washington, DC: American Psychiatric Press, 1996: 235–263.
70. Hendrie HC, Callahan CM, Levitt EE, Hui SL, Musick B, Austrom MG, Nurnberger JI, Jr., Tierney WM. Prevalence rates of major depressive disorders: The effects of varying the diagnostic criteria in an older primary care population. American Journal of Geriatric Psychiatry 1995; 3: 119–131.

71. Lam R, Pacala J, Smith S. Factors related to depressive symptoms in an elderly Chinese American sample. Clinical Gerontologist 1997; 17: 57–70.
72. Mui AC. Depression among elderly Chinese immigrants: An exploratory study. Social Work 1996; 41: 633–645.
73. Mui AC. Stress, coping, and depression among elderly Korean immigrants. Journal of Human Behavior in the Social Environment 2001; 3: 281–299.
74. Zhang AY, Yu LC, Yuan J, Tong A, Yang C, Foreman SE. Family and cultural correlates of depression among Chinese elderly. International Journal of Social Psychiatry 1997; 43: 199–212.
75. Stokes SC, Thompson LW, Murphy S. Screening for depression in immigrant Chinese-American elders: Results of a pilot study. Journal of Gerontological Social Work 2001; 36: 27–44.
76. Wu B, Tran TV, Amjad Q. Chronic illnesses and depression among Chinese immigrant elders. Journal of Gerontological Social Work 2004; 43: 79–95.
77. Yamamoto J, Rhee S, Chang DS. Psychiatric disorders among elderly Koreans in the United States. Community Mental Health Journal 1994; 30: 17–27.
78. Carney SS, Rich CL, Burke PA, Fowler RC. Suicide over 60: The San Diego Study. Journal of the American Geriatrics Society 1994; 42: 174–180.
79. Yu ES. Health of the Chinese elderly in America. Research on Aging 1986; 8: 84–109.
80. Bui KT, Takeuchi DT. Ethnic minority adolescents and the use of community mental health care services. American Journal of Community Psychology 1992; 20: 403–418.
81. Chen S, Sullivan NY, Lu YE, Shibusawa T. Asian Americans and mental health services: A study of utilization patterns in the 1990s. Journal of Ethnic Cultural Diversity in Social Work 2003; 12: 19–42.
82. Cheung FK, Snowden LR. Community mental health and ethnic minority populations. Community Mental Health Journal 1990; 26: 277–291.
83. Zhang AY, Snowden LR, Sue S. Differences between Asian and White Americans' help seeking and utilization patterns in the Los Angeles area. Journal of Community Psychology 1998; 26: 317–326.
84. Matsuoka JK, Breaux C, Ryujin DH. National utilization of mental health services by Asian Americans/Pacific Islanders. Journal of Community Psychology 1997; 25: 141–145.
85. Sue S. Community mental health services to minority groups: Some optimism, some pessimism. American Psychologist 1977; 32: 616–624.
86. Sue DW, Sue D. Counseling the culturally different. New York: Wiley, 1999.
87. Wong EC, Marshall GN, Schell TL, Elliott MN, Hambarsoomians K, Chun C, Berthold SM. Barriers to mental health care utilization for U.S. Cambodian refugees. Journal of Consulting & Clinical Psychology 2006; 74:1116–1120.

Assessing Asian American Family Acculturation in Clinical Settings: Guidelines and Recommendations for Mental Health Professionals

K. M. Chun and P. D. Akutsu

Abstract In this chapter, we present the background and rationale for assessing acculturation in Asian American families. We discuss key Asian American family acculturation issues: family dynamics, family structure, developmental considerations, and family ecologies. In addition, we present clinical guidelines to assess Asian American family acculturation and its impact on the parent–child and couple subsystems.

Keywords Family acculturation · Asian American family therapy · Family dynamics · Family ecologies · Family structure · Parent–child subsystem · Couple subsystem

Contents
Key Asian American Family Acculturation Issues............................ 101
   Family Dynamics 102
   Family Structure 103
   Developmental Considerations... 103
   Family Ecologies... 104
Special Focus on Assessing Acculturation in Parent–Child and Couple Subsystems . 106
   Assessing Acculturation Issues in the Parent–Child Subsystem 106
   Assessing Acculturation Issues in the Couple Subsystem 112
Conclusion 117
References... 119

Significant advancements in acculturation research over the past two decades have shed new light on the psychological implications of immigration, relocation, and resettlement for the growing number of Asian immigrants entering the United States. In particular, the development of new acculturation measures

---

K.M. Chun (✉)
Department of Psychology, University of San Francisco, 2130 Fulton Street, San Francisco, CA 94117-1080, USA
e-mail: chunk@usfca.edu

provides rich opportunities for group-specific acculturation analyses [1], comparative multiethnic group analyses [2, 3], and focused analyses of selected acculturation domains [4, 5]. In addition, important linkages between acculturation and mental health have been established; acculturation stress generally increases risk for depressive and anxiety symptoms [6–9], but certain protective factors (e.g., social support, younger age, and knowledge of the United States prior to immigration) guard against acculturation stress and psychosocial dysfunction [10]. Lastly, conceptual and theoretical advancements in acculturation research have highlighted the multidimensional and dynamic properties of acculturation, sparking reformulations of and improvements to early linear acculturation models that posited an inevitable loss of cultural behaviors and traits with culture contact [11].

Collectively, these developments in acculturation measurement, research, and theory have encouraged mental health professionals to more fully consider how acculturation affects the psychological adjustment of their Asian American clients. The formal inclusion of "acculturation stress" as a psychosocial stressor in the DSM-IV further encourages acculturation assessment in clinical evaluation and diagnosis. Still, clinicians and other mental health service providers are confronted with a number of practical constraints and challenges in assessing their clients' acculturation. This is perhaps most evident when attempting to evaluate Asian American immigrant families in clinical or therapeutic settings. To date, most acculturation instruments and measures for Asian Americans were primarily developed for research purposes using college student populations; thus, their utility and appropriateness for clinical assessment with new immigrants (particularly for those with little formal education and low English proficiency) are not always clear or might prove to be impractical or unfeasible. In this latter case, some self-report measures might be too lengthy or time-consuming for intake interviews and clinical assessment and some are not readily available in various Asian languages. Acculturation measures for Asian Americans also tend to focus on individual acculturation experiences, making it difficult for mental health professionals to comprehend the family context of acculturation. Most self-report acculturation measures focus on either individual background characteristics (e.g., birthplace, years of residency in the United States, English language proficiency) or individual cultural traits and behaviors (e.g., individual cultural socialization experiences, food/music/clothing preferences, and individual attitudes and beliefs) rather than on family acculturation experiences. Thus, clinicians often lack a clear and comprehensive means to directly evaluate complex acculturation processes in Asian Americans families and their significance to overall family functioning.

Assessing acculturation at the family level is an important consideration for several reasons. First, recently arrived Asian American immigrants are more likely to live in multigenerational or extended family households. According to a 2002 US Census report, approximately 73% of Asian Americans come from family rather than from non-family households, and around one out of every five married–coupled Asian American households report five or more family members [12]. Acculturation among Asian American immigrants is thus more likely to occur in a family rather than in an individual or isolated context. Second, the family is a central component of daily life for those Asian American immigrants who possess a collectivistic social orientation and family-oriented cultural values (e.g., family obligation, respect for elders). Collectivistic concerns about family well-being and cultural expectations to attend to family rather than to individual needs invariably frame and organize new immigrants' daily activities, including how they navigate a new cultural environment and cope with acculturation stress. Finally, family systems, structural family therapy, and family ecology models propose that individual psychosocial adjustment is intimately related to overall family functioning [13]. Thus, individual adjustment and adaptation to a new cultural setting can likewise be shaped by family context, including family dynamics or family relations, family structure or family organization, family development, and the characteristics of family ecologies.

A primary goal of this chapter is to provide mental health professionals with practical guidelines and recommendations to assess acculturation in Asian American immigrant families in clinical or therapy settings. To this end, the chapter is organized into two main sections that, respectively, focus on (a) identifying key family acculturation issues and stressors that influence Asian American family functioning and (b) outlining practical interview questions that allow clinicians to assess these family acculturation issues during intake and therapy sessions. Assessing acculturation issues in the parent–child and couple subsystems will be the focus of this second section because much of the acculturation literature on Asian American families concentrates on these two family groupings. For the purposes of this chapter, we offer the following working definition of acculturation:

> A dynamic and multidimensional process of adaptation and adjustment that occurs with sustained contact between distinct cultures. It involves different degrees and instances of cultural learning, maintenance, and synthesis that are contingent upon individual, group, and environmental factors. Acculturation is dynamic because it is a continuous and fluctuating process, and it is multidimensional because it transpires across multiple indices of psychosocial functioning.

The following section illustrates how the multidimensional and dynamic nature of acculturation is fully expressed in Asian American families.

Key Asian American Family Acculturation Issues

The complexities of family acculturation are revealed when considering how acculturation can vary with family dynamics, family structures, the developmental tasks and skills of individual members, and family ecologies [14]. In the following section, the significance of these areas of family functioning to acculturation is reviewed in the context of family systems, structural family therapy, and family ecology frameworks.

Family Dynamics

Acculturation can be influenced by family dynamics or the ways in which family members relate to one another. According to family systems theory, family relations are interdependent or "hard-wired" together such that the actions of one family member potentially influence those of other members [13, 15]. The acculturation experiences of Asian American family members can thus be "hard-wired" together – the nature and rate of acculturation of one member can potentially affect the acculturation experiences of other members [16]. For instance, older siblings can hasten their younger siblings' acculturation by deciphering and transmitting new cultural knowledge and skills to them in their role as a "cultural broker" [17]. Conversely, rates of family acculturation can be inhibited or slowed by a family member; an older family member, for instance, may discourage other family members from bringing new cultural skills and beliefs into the family system, thus limiting how the entire family learns about and responds to a new culture.

Acculturation can also be affected by the tempo at which Asian American families function. During acculturation, immigrant families might be pressed to change or adjust the rhythm of their daily routines to match the pace and time orientation in a new culture. According to Sue and Sue [18], dominant American culture promotes a "future" time orientation evidenced by its emphasis on youth and achievement, controlling one's destiny, planning for the future, and maintaining an optimistic and hopeful future outlook. This future time orientation presents some challenges to Asian American families who follow a "past–present" orientation that links family history and reverence for the past (e.g., respecting family ancestors) with their present day lives and activities, and treats age as a marker of wisdom, respectability, and authority. Asian American families may experience acculturation stress when attempting to reconcile these two conflicting time orientations. For example, older Asian immigrants may face considerable acculturation stress when younger family members adopt an American future time orientation that diminishes their authority and decision-making powers that were traditionally afforded to them in their culture of origin.

Lastly, the extent to which Asian American family members expand or transform the ways in which they relate to one another in a new cultural environment can also affect their collective experience of acculturation. New life challenges, including those imposed by immigration and relocation, typically require family members to achieve greater flexibility in their family relations or to develop entirely new ways of interacting with one another. When families follow customary or familiar interaction patterns that are no longer effective in a new cultural environment, they can enter a state of "homeostasis" in which they essentially become "stuck" during their acculturation process [14]. Asian American immigrant parents who might have effectively communicated with their children using unidirectional or one-way communication may encounter acculturation difficulties when faced with new cultural norms favoring bidirectional parent–child communication or mutual dialog and negotiation. If new or modified communication patterns are not established, then homeostasis and resultant acculturation stress can subsequently arise in the parent–child subsystem.

Family Structure

Asian American family structure, or the ways families organize themselves, is another important consideration in family acculturation. According to structural family therapy, family members form distinct groupings or subsystems based on characteristic patterns of family interactions [19]. Asian American families can exhibit a broad range of subsystems in multigenerational households, each with its own culturally prescribed family roles and expectations for behaviors, reflecting their cultural values and beliefs, social orientation, and socioeconomic needs and resources. Consequently, Asian American family subsystems can include family groupings associated with nuclear households (e.g., parent–child, couple, and sibling subsystems) in addition to other culturally meaningful subsystems that extend beyond Western definitions of the family (e.g., generational, task-oriented, and gender subsystems; grandparents or extended family members serving as primary caregivers in a parenting subsystem). The implications of diverse family constellations for Asian American family acculturation are quite significant when considering that acculturation experiences, including the types of acculturation stressors that family members encounter, can vary across these different family groupings. As such, there can be highly varied and constantly fluctuating acculturation experiences within a single-family unit, necessitating multiple reference points for acculturation assessment.

Acculturation rates can also vary for individual family members as they move in and out of different family subsystems. For instance, a wife may acculturate at a faster rate in the couple subsystem (e.g., by resisting traditional gender role expectations in her marriage), yet acculturate at a slower rate in the parent–child subsystem (e.g., by insisting that her children respect her role as a maternal authority figure). Similarly, a family member's rate of acculturation can vary across gender subsystems. For instance, studies have found that male Asian American family members are often afforded more freedom and independence in exploring extrafamilial environments, allowing them more opportunities than their female counterparts to acquire new cultural information and skills [20, 21].

Developmental Considerations

Asian American family acculturation is also intimately tied to the developmental skills and tasks of family members. Given that acculturation fundamentally involves acquiring, maintaining, and synthesizing cultural information and behaviors, these processes will vary according to family members' age-related differences in cognitive, language, interpersonal skills and abilities, and life experiences. In addition, their different developmental tasks potentially influence what they find most stressful during acculturation, in many respects framing their perception and experience of acculturation stress. From an Eriksonian perspective, Asian American adolescent immigrants may be particularly concerned with identity formation issues during acculturation; hence, establishing a clear reference group of peers in their new cultural environment may be an especially salient acculturation stressor. Their elderly grandparents, however, might experience an entirely different set of acculturation stressors; concerns over constructing meaning in their lives may be their most salient acculturation issue, thus maintaining or reestablishing purposeful and meaningful roles in their family and community may be a primary source of acculturation stress.

The developmental context of acculturation therefore represents a key consideration in assessing the overall functioning of immigrant Asian American families. A structural family therapy framework underscores the importance of evaluating the life cycles of family functioning. According to this framework, families are in a continuous process of change involving periods of adaptation and balance (involving mastery of skills) and instances of disequilibrium (arising from individual members or from changing contexts) [22]. In terms of family acculturation assessment, this is a useful framework to conceptualize how a family's stage of acculturation might be linked to specific acculturation concerns. This framework can likewise help mental health professionals determine where and how to "join" with an Asian American immigrant family at the outset of therapy: Is the family in a state of disequilibrium in their acculturation process requiring the therapist to provide clarity to their life circumstances? What are the structural underpinnings of the family's current state of disequilibrium – that is, what are the specific family roles that they are struggling to enact, and how might this be related to their presenting acculturation difficulties? Or is the family entering a stage of adaptation and balance in their acculturation process? If so, are they primarily seeking help and reassurance to expand their repertoire of behaviors so that they can progress toward a new and more complex phase of family functioning?

Family Ecologies

Family members potentially move through a multitude of family ecologies throughout the course of their daily lives, with each presenting a unique set of conditions for cultural learning, maintenance, and synthesis. According to a family ecology model, parents can inhabit different extrafamilial adult ecologies or "exosystems," which can include their work settings and adult social circles, while their children and youth move through different extrafamilial youth ecologies or "mesosystems," such as their school and peer group settings [23]. Acculturation experiences, including levels of acculturation stress, can vary across Asian American family members given that each faces a different set of acculturation demands in these extrafamilial ecologies. Moreover, family members can share newly acquired cultural knowledge from these extrafamilial ecologies, which can expand their collective ability to adapt to new cultural contexts. Conversely, new cultural information from these extrafamilial ecologies can push families into a state of disequilibrium by eliciting family conflict and acculturation stress.

Ethnic minority status is another important ecological consideration in Asian American family acculturation [24, 25]. Not only do Asian American families face acculturation demands to learn, maintain, and synthesize cultural information and skills but also they must do so in a racially stratified society. Newer immigrants who have never been exposed to racial prejudice and discrimination in their countries of origin and are unaware of the complicated legacy of race in the United States might be especially confused or shocked by this experience. Sue and Sue [18] assert that acculturation in the United States should therefore be conceptualized as an interaction between dominant and minority groups. These authors believe that acculturation stress arising from intergenerational conflict is a manifestation of larger societal pressures for ethnic minorities to adopt dominant group cultural norms. Mental health professionals should therefore assess the racial context of Asian American family acculturation, which can include evaluating a family's exposure to racism, the ethnic and cultural characteristics of their community, their overall awareness of racial issues, and the ways in which they cope with ethnic minority status during acculturation.

Lastly, the effects of transnational family ecologies on Asian American family acculturation are becoming more palpable given the expansion of globalization, transnational migration, and international cultural exchange over the past decade [26]. Acculturation processes can begin prior to actual migration with exposure to new cultural information through the media, commercial exchange, and contact with family and friends who reside in the United States. Upon resettlement, immigrants with sufficient financial means may also traverse and reside in various countries (e.g., maintaining dual residences or staying with family and friends in Asia and in the United States for extended periods). This type of transnational movement can help families maintain their cultural practices, including maintaining their culturally prescribed family roles. In short, the timing, space, and location in which family acculturation transpires is radically shifting with increasing transnationalism and globalization; thus, acculturation models and assessment tools that frame acculturation as a discrete, postmigration phenomenon need to be revised. Family acculturation assessment can address this issue by attending to the potential effects of transnational Asian American family activities and networks on overall family adaptation in the United States.

Special Focus on Assessing Acculturation in Parent–Child and Couple Subsystems

Acculturation effects on parent–child and couple relations continue to garner significant attention in the Asian American family acculturation literature [26]. This section thus provides an overview of key acculturation issues in both of these family subsystems. Furthermore, this section is specifically tailored to mental health professionals who are interested in practical interview questions that will help them to assess these key issues during intake or therapy. The assessment interview questions outlined below are intended to address the complexities of family acculturation and functioning that are not fully captured by traditional individual self-report measures. Detailed instruction on how to present these questions in a culturally appropriate manner, including advice on conducting culturally competent clinical interviews as well as assessment and therapy, can be found in a growing body of ethnic minority psychology scholarship on these topics (e.g., 18, 27, 28).

Assessing Acculturation Issues in the Parent–Child Subsystem

Conflict over Family Practices and Values

Asian American immigrant family practices are often informed by Confucian family hierarchies, with family members assigned to well-defined roles based on age, role, sex, and birth order [29, 30]. Typically, the father or grandfather wields the most power in family decisions, while the mother provides nurturance and support to the children. Older siblings, especially the eldest daughter, are often delegated childcare responsibilities for younger siblings and are expected to assist their mothers with household duties (e.g., cooking, cleaning). Asian American immigrant parents may also place a higher value on sons over daughters, expecting the oldest son in particular to support them during their senior years, and to act as stewards for younger siblings throughout their lives. Regardless of gender or age, Asian American immigrant parents often expect their children to be obedient, hardworking, and respectful of their authority and to place family needs above their own.

In contrast to this Asian family structure, American cultural family practices and values emphasize independence, self-reliance, autonomy, assertiveness, open dialog, and competition [29, 30]. These types of values are often more attractive to Asian American children who may then seek to introduce them into their immigrant households. Research has shown that Asian American children might acculturate faster than their immigrant parents to such American beliefs, leading to parent–child conflicts over restrictive family roles, career goals, dating, and marriage [31, 30].

In response to increasing acculturation in their children, Asian American immigrant parents may exert more restrictions on their children's activities.

For example, immigrant parents may become even more involved in their children's decisions about education (e.g., enrolling them in afterschool Asian language programs, guiding their selection of colleges and majors) and place greater barriers on nonacademic extracurricular activities (e.g., socializing with friends, dating). Often, immigrant parents apply such pressures with the hope of fostering greater cultural commitment in their children, yet these actions often drive their children further away from embracing traditional Asian family values [32]. The few studies on family dynamics, ethnic identity, and acculturation suggest that feelings of ethnic pride are more likely to occur in immigrant families that are marked by warmth and independence [33] and supportive family relations may be a vital prerequisite for exploration and retention of one's culture of origin among minority youth [34]. While past studies show that Asian American immigrant parents are more likely to engage in controlling parenting styles than European American parents [26], acculturation can lead to less-controlling child-rearing attitudes in Asian American families over time [35–38]. The following questions can be asked to assess parent–child acculturation conflict issues:

- Since moving to the United States, have you noticed any changes in who makes important decisions for your family? Who has the power of authority and how are decision-making and tasks accomplished in your family?
- How are family responsibilities, rules, and expectations communicated in your family? Has this changed since moving to the United States?
- Since moving to the United States, have there been any shifts in your parents'/children's roles, behaviors, and attitudes? If so, to what do you attribute these changes?
- Ideally, what should be the roles, duties, and responsibilities of parents and children? Do your parents/children act in this way in your own family? Has this changed since moving to the United States?

Conflict over Communication and Emotional Expression

Asian American children sometimes complain about the lack of warmth and open communication in their relationships with their parents. Although the importance of interdependence is emphasized in Asian American immigrant families, the manner in which caring is expressed to children and other family members is often through instrumental support (e.g., helping with homework, preparing special meals) rather than emotional support (e.g., open displays of affection, hugging). In some Asian cultures, parents believe that open displays of affection can be too demonstrative and are unnecessary for their children's development [30, 39]. Although Asian American immigrant parents can be physically affectionate to very young children, cultural pressures to reduce such behaviors begin as early as the preschool years and physical signs of affection steadily diminish after that age period. However, as Asian American children see how their peers from other ethnic groups engage with their parents, they may begin to prefer more open parent–child communication and emotional displays. Many Asian American immigrant parents do not openly praise their children because they feel that this could inflate their ego and discourage them from remaining focused in their academic studies. As such, Asian American children might interpret their parents' behavior as a sign of disapproval or a lack of parental love and acceptance.

Regarding communication in traditional Asian American immigrant families, there is a tendency to follow unidirectional communication, where the flow of communication occurs along a family hierarchy – from husband to wife, parents to children, and older siblings to younger siblings. These traditional communication patterns are established to ensure clear family role boundaries and to avoid direct questioning of family power dynamics. These types of communication practices, however, may be viewed as excessively rigid in comparison with European American communication patterns where the family might be more open to dissenting opinions before a final decision is made. Asian American children often become aware of these types of egalitarian communication patterns in their schools where open debate and sharing ideas are reinforced. Again, as Asian American children become more acculturated, they may interpret their parents' unwillingness to allow them to become more active in family decisions as a sign of distrust in their opinions.

In response, many Asian American children may turn to alternative sources of support such as spending more time at non-Asian American friends' homes or developing bonds with teachers or other adult figures to receive open praise that they perceive to be lacking in their homes. Parent–child conflict can arise in these situations when Asian American immigrant parents question the motives of these non-family members and subsequently enforce greater restrictions on their children. Parents may attribute these conflict issues to their children's increasing acculturation, but these issues may reflect normative developmental tasks for youth as they seek greater autonomy, particularly during adolescence. The tendency of Asian American immigrant parents to label their children's acculturation as a sign of assimilation indicates that they may view it as a threatening process that invariably disrupts and imbalances the parent–child subsystem. The following questions can be presented to both parents and their children to evaluate their conflict over communication:

- How do you and your child/parent talk and communicate with each other? In your mind, how should parents and children ideally communicate with each other?
- Do you see differences in how parents and their children communicate here in the United States versus how parents and their children communicate in your culture of origin? What are these differences? What types of challenges do these differences present?
- How do you express your concerns and feelings to each other? Since moving to the United States, has this changed? If so, in what ways has this challenged

or improved your relationship? How do you think these changes in your communication happened?
- Do you feel that it is appropriate in your culture to openly express emotions in the family? Why or why not?

Differential Experiences of Acculturation

Recent studies illustrate that Asian American parents and their children may experience acculturation differently. Immigrant parents tend to view acculturation as a unidimensional process; thus increased acculturation is perceived to invariably weaken attachment to traditional Asian values. In contrast, Asian American children who view themselves as being bicultural see movement toward American cultural values as a separate process that does not affect their identification with Asian cultural values [4, 40]. These different perceptions of acculturation can therefore spark conflict in the parent–child subsystem.

Asian American immigrant parents may also feel ambivalent about their children's acculturation concerns because they are unaware of the difficulties that their children face in negotiating different cultural identities in their daily lives. For example, parents may expect their children be quiet, obedient, and respectful in their homes, yet fail to comprehend that certain behaviors learned during acculturation, such as increased assertiveness, initiative, and independent thinking, are necessary for success in American schools and society [41]. This often places great pressures on Asian American children as they struggle to manage these different cultural demands and expectations. While Asian American immigrant parents want their children to quickly develop strong English skills and master certain American practices for success in the classroom, they may also require their children to participate in afterschool or weekend Asian language schools to ensure that they learn about Asian cultural traditions. These types of parental practices that are intended to counteract their children's acculturation to US culture can generate parent–child conflict.

As a therapist working with Asian American families, understanding differences in how parents and their children experience acculturation can provide insights to underlying factors in Asian American parent–child conflicts. For immigrant parents, acculturation might be seen as a threat to positive Asian values, symbolizing a negation or rejection of Asian customs by their children. Bicultural Asian American youth might feel dumbstruck that their immigrant parents are making such a fuss because from their perspective acculturation does not affect their attachment to their Asian cultural heritage. Although both parents and children might acknowledge that movement toward American culture is clearly visible for Asian American youth, their interpretations of this movement can thus be quite different. To assess differential experiences of acculturation in the parent–child subsystem, the following questions can be presented. As Asian American parents and children may have different perspectives and feelings about the topics of these questions, it may be best to ask them in separate sessions to ensure greater disclosure.

Parents

- Do you feel that moving to this country has changed family members' identification with and attachment to your cultural group?
- What Asian cultural values do you want your children to learn? Why do you want them to learn these values? Do you feel that they can learn about American cultural values at the same time? Why or why not?
- Are you concerned that your children are becoming "too American?" In what ways do you think your children have become "too American?" What have you said or done to try to stop this from happening? Has it worked?

Children

- Do you feel that moving to this country has changed family members' identification with and attachment to your cultural group?
- What American cultural values do you want your parents to learn? Why do you want them to learn these values? Do you feel that they can learn and adopt more American cultural values? Why or why not?
- Do your parents feel like you are becoming "too American?" What have they said or done to communicate this to you? How have you responded to their comments? Do you believe that you are becoming more American? What does this mean to you?

Role Reversals

Role reversals in the parent–child subsystem can occur when children possess more cultural skills than their parents and acculturation demands press them to serve as "cultural brokers" or "language brokers" for their parents in extra-familial ecologies [42, 43]. Many Asian American immigrant parents are severely restricted in their ability to interface with social institutions (e.g., schools, medical and legal systems) outside of their homes and ethnic enclaves because of their limited English fluency and lack of cultural knowledge about these institutions. If Asian American children acculturate faster than their immigrant parents, they are likely to become more proficient in English and possess more bicultural competencies. Recent studies show that more than 75% of Asian American adolescents (Chinese, Korean, and Vietnamese American) have language brokered for their immigrant families [44, 43]. Although first-generation Asian American adolescents reported the highest percentages of language brokering, second-generation Asian American adolescents also reported high levels of brokering (57% for Chinese American and 67% for Korean American second-generation adolescents) [44].

Some clinicians have cautioned that parents should not rely on their children to fulfill important family duties because it potentially leads to "childhood parentification," which can compromise family dynamics and adolescent development [44, 45]. Such dependence between immigrant parents and their children might evoke resentment in both parties and increase the likelihood of disagreements and conflict. However, the relatively few studies that have examined psychological consequences of cultural brokering for Asian American youth have reported mixed findings. Some studies have reported positive rather than negative feelings about cultural brokering for Asian American adolescents and their families [43]. Chao [44] recently found interesting differences across Asian ethnic groups and family members in this latter regard – cultural brokering increased Korean American youths' respect for their fathers and heightened Chinese American youths' respect for their mothers. In this same study, however, cultural brokering was associated with greater internalizing and externalizing psychological symptoms for these same Korean American youth and more internalizing psychological problems for these Chinese American youth. These findings suggest that cultural brokering in diverse Asian American immigrant families remains a complex issue involving multiple dimensions of family dynamics (e.g., family communication and family expectations) and perhaps culture-specific socialization and parenting practices. In studying Latino families, researchers caution that cultural brokering is often "taken-for-granted household work," and clinicians should be cautious about placing too much importance on these duties [46–48].

The following questions can be asked to assess role reversals and its effects on the parent–child subsystem. Because Asian American parents or children may have different feelings and concerns about cultural brokering, these questions should be presented to them in separate interviews [30, 49].

Parents

- How often does your child act as an English language translator for you and your family? How often does your child help you to complete daily chores or family duties that require English translations? With what types of activities does he/she assist you and other family members?
- How have these translating activities affected your relationship with your child?
- How does it make you feel to ask your son or daughter to translate or do these things for you?

Children

- How often do you or your siblings act as an English language translator for your parents and your family? How often do you or your siblings help your parents or other family members to complete daily chores that require English translations? With what types of activities do you or your siblings assist your parents and other family members?
- How have these translating activities affected your relationship with your parents and other family members?
- How do you feel about translating or interpreting things for your parents and other family members?

Significance of Exosystems and Mesosystems to Parent–Child Acculturation

Many Asian American children and adolescents observe cultural differences in their upbringing through their social interactions in different "mesosytems" or extrafamilial youth ecologies, such as their schools and peer groups [23]. As they begin to adopt more American values and behaviors from these mesosystems, Asian American immigrant parents may feel threatened by this. However, parents may come to embrace certain aspects of the American lifestyle from their different "exosystems" or extrafamilial adult ecologies, such as their work settings and adult social circles. "Cultural conflict" may occur when one spouse is more acculturated than the other, which could then impact the parent–child relationship with subsequent shifts in their discipline practices, parental expectations, and family communication patterns. For example, cultural conflict can occur if a husband holds onto to his traditional family role, whereas his wife and children adopt more acculturated egalitarian family relationships. Parent–child acculturation in Asian American families can thus be facilitated or complicated by exposure to extrafamilial ecologies, although mere exposure to these ecologies does not necessarily lead to rapid acculturation changes in the parent–child subsystem. Rather, acculturation shifts are often subtle, occurring over long periods of time with gradual and reciprocal exchanges of cultural information between parents, children, and their respective ecologies. To assess the significance of extrafamilial ecologies to parent–child acculturation, the following questions can be asked:

- To what extent do you interact with and socialize with people outside of your home? What have you learned about American culture from these people? Have they changed your beliefs about what it means to be a family, including changing your beliefs about the roles and duties of parents and children, and how parents and children should interact and communicate with each other?
- How do you interact with each other at home? Do feel like your interactions are different from how you see other parents and children interacting with each other? What do you make of these differences? Do you feel the need to change how you interact and communicate with each other based on these differences?

Assessing Acculturation Issues in the Couple Subsystem

Shifts in Gender Attitudes and Roles

As Asian American couples resettle in a new culture, spouses can experience differential rates of acculturation that can catalyze shifts in their gender roles. Acculturation experiences can vary in the couple subsystem with differential exposure to new cultural information between spouses. For instance, an immigrant wife might possess a greater repertoire of cultural skills than her husband (e.g., greater English language proficiency and more culturally relevant job skills), which gives her greater access to new cultural information across diverse extrafamilial ecologies. New cultural information can include new cultural norms about gender role expectations that may compel some Asian American immigrant women to reevaluate their cultural beliefs about marriage. The couple subsystem can become imbalanced by acculturation pressures that alter how spouses function in their relationship particularly if both spouses had agreed earlier upon the culturally prescribed gender roles of their country of origin. For Asian American women, shifts in gender attitudes can elicit acculturation stress as they attempt to negotiate conflicting cultural expectations and roles at home and work [20, 21]. To assess possible shifts in gender attitudes and roles during acculturation the following questions can be asked:

- Have your roles as a husband and wife changed since moving to the United States? If so, how have your roles changed and how has this affected your current relationship?
- How do you divide your daily family and household responsibilities in your marriage and family? What "works" and "does not work" for you with this arrangement?
- What are your expectations for one another in your relationship? Have these expectations changed since moving to the United States? What types of challenges have you faced in trying to meet these relationship expectations in the United States?
- In your culture, what are the expected duties of husbands and wives? Do you believe that the duties of husbands and wives are different in America? Have these cultural differences in duties caused you any problems in your relationship or family?

Status Inconsistency

Status inconsistency can co-occur with shifting gender roles when a spouse experiences a loss of occupational, economic, social, and family status and prestige following immigration. Much of the literature on this topic indicates that Asian American immigrant men are more likely than Asian American women to experience status inconsistency given the presence of patriarchal family structures and social roles that privilege men in Asia [20]. Status inconsistency issues were poignantly displayed in a study of Southeast Asian veterans of the Vietnam War who relocated to the United States [50]. A former Vietnamese general in this study who once commanded 10,000 troops across several South Vietnamese provinces was forced to retrain as a social worker in the United States because he could not find gainful employment as a military professional. Although he was able to provide for his family's basic needs as a social worker, he experienced tremendous shame and loss of face because he could no longer bring the same prestige to his family as he had once done in Vietnam. He thus felt depressed, anxious, and emotionally detached from his wife and family believing that he had "failed" in his roles as a husband, father, and military leader. Status inconsistency issues in the couple subsystem can be assessed by the following questions:

- Did your social, occupational, or family status change when you moved to the United States? Can you please tell me about these changes? How have you and your spouse coped with these changes?
- As a couple, how would you describe the quality of your life in your country of origin? Is life harder or more difficult for both of you in the United States? Can you tell me what changes have made it more difficult for you? How has this affected your relationship together?
- What was your job in your country of origin? Is it different from your current job? If you have changed jobs, which job do you prefer? Why?
- Do you feel that your family, friends, and co-workers still view and treat you the same way here in the United States as they did in your country of origin?
- Have changes to your social, occupational, and family status in the United States affected your ability to fulfill your responsibilities as a husband/wife or family provider/head of household?

Changes in Couple Dynamics and Risk for Domestic Abuse

When spousal roles are realigned during acculturation, parallel changes in couple dynamics can occur. For instance, decision-making authority and power in the marriage can be contested and redistributed between spouses, which can affect their communication, marital satisfaction, and sense of intimacy. An immigrant wife who assumes a new role of primary provider for her household may desire a more egalitarian marital relationship. However, if her husband insists on maintaining familiar patriarchal gender roles, their couple subsystem may enter a state of homeostasis and become "stuck" during acculturation if they cannot effectively negotiate their new couple roles, boundaries, and ways of functioning. In such circumstances, acculturation can lead to marital conflict, emotional distancing between spouses, dissolution of the couple subsystem, or, in the worst-case scenario, domestic violence. Minuchin and Fishman [22] offered commentary on couple dynamics that captures the potential pressures that acculturation imposes on the couple subsystem, particularly when spouses struggle to negotiate and incorporate new cultural expectations and behaviors in their relationship:

> "...if the rules of the subsystem are so rigid that the experiences gained by each spouse in extrafamilial transactions cannot be incorporated, the 'spouses in the subsystem' may be bound to inadequate survival rules by past contracts and allowed a more diversified use of self only when away from each other. In this situation, the spouse subsystem will grow more and more impoverished, and devitalized, ultimately becoming unavailable as a source of growth for its members. If these conditions continue, the spouses may find it necessary to dismantle the subsystem (pp. 16–17)."

In this context, acculturation demands can reveal implicit and explicit rules and assumptions that govern a couple's relationship. The extent to which each spouse is willing and able to reformulate these rules and assumptions will determine whether they can grow and become a more flexible and expansive subsystem during acculturation. The interdependent nature of couple acculturation suggests that spouses can actively facilitate or even hinder each other during this process. In the worst circumstances, domestic violence can occur if a spouse approaches acculturation demands from a position of diminished authority or low self-esteem [51, 52]. In addition, cultural norms that privilege male authority and ascribe secondary status to women in the couple subsystem increase risk for domestic violence during acculturation [53, 54]. Pertinent assessment questions regarding acculturation effects on couple dynamics and consequent risks for domestic violence include the following (these questions can be presented to individual spouses in separate sessions):

- Have you changed the ways that you relate to and communicate with one another since moving to the United States? How have these changes affected your relationship? How have these changes affected how you have adjusted to the United States as a couple?
- Have you asked your spouse to make any changes in your relationship since moving to the United States? How did he/she respond to this request?
- Has moving to the United States created conflict in your relationship? What types of conflict have you experienced since moving to the United States? How do you handle these conflicts as a couple?
- Do you feel that your spouse supports your effort to adjust to American culture? What does he/she do to support you? What do you wish he/she would do differently to help support you?
- Does your spouse help you to maintain your cultural traditions? What does he/she do?

Developmental Acculturation Concerns

The developmental context of acculturation in Asian American couples is another important consideration. The couple subsystem, like other family subsystems, experiences different stages of growth characterized by periods of crisis, change, and transition. The ways in which couples respond to new life challenges are shaped by their shared history, life perspective, and how well spouses have come to know one another, including how well they know each other's strengths and limitations. Older couples with considerable life experience together have had more opportunities to synchronize their behaviors to meet life's challenges, and may respond differently to acculturation demands than younger couples. Still, this does not mean that older couples are less susceptible to acculturation stress; rather, age and development help to frame how couples experience acculturation. For instance, a couple's acculturation issues may reflect their unique developmental concerns and tasks. For older couples, developmental concerns about the meaning and purpose of their lives in their late adulthood may frame their acculturation experience. Acculturation issues pertaining to diminished family roles, loss of social and family support systems, isolation and loneliness, and a fear of becoming a burden to family members might therefore be particularly salient to them [55–58]. These types of acculturation concerns can become even more distressing if these couples face health problems or lack economic resources and cultural skills that prevent them from maintaining active family and social roles. These types of developmental considerations in couple acculturation can be evaluated with the following questions:

- How long have you been together as a couple? Do you feel like the time that you have spent together affects how you handle life challenges as a couple? Have your life experiences together influenced your ability to adjust to life in the United States?
- Some people say that couples grow and mature over time and enter different stages in their relationship. How would you describe the stage of your relationship that you are in right now? Do you think that this has influenced your ability to resettle in the United States together?
- What have you learned about each other during the course of your relationship? How has this affected your ability to work together or get along with one another in this country?
- At this time in your lives, what are you most concerned about as a couple? Have these concerns influenced how you are currently experiencing your life together in the United States?

Ecological Factors in Couple Acculturation

Ecological factors such as ethnic minority status and transnational family ecologies can also influence acculturation experiences in the Asian American couple subsystem. Asian American immigrant couples may have to learn how to cope with prejudice and discrimination in a racially stratified society, and immigrant women may have to contend with the added stressor of sexism. Prejudice and discrimination can be especially disconcerting for new immigrant couples who are unfamiliar with historical racial paradigms and hierarchies in the United States. For these couples, the unfortunate realities of racial oppression in contemporary American society potentially compound the stress of reestablishing a new life in this country. A couple's cultural resources such as their family and community support networks, religious organizations, and other forms of social capital can buffer the negative effects of acculturation stress associated with ethnic minority status [59]. Transnational activities and family networks can likewise serve as important protective factors for couple acculturation; Asian American couples who receive emotional and instrumental support from their family and social circles abroad, spend extended periods of time returning to and staying in their countries of origin, and maintain positive social roles in their countries of origin (e.g., spouses who maintain their role as a valued community, church, or business leader, being a respected member in a Chinese family association) can nurture their cultural identities and become more resilient to race-related stressors in the United States. Transnational activities that link couples with their cultures of origin can also support cultural maintenance in the couple subsystem (e.g., the maintenance of culturally prescribed gender roles) and provide opportunities for cultural synthesis or the development of bicultural identities. Asian American couple acculturation should thus be assessed with a broad lens to capture the expanding transnational social spheres in which it unfolds. The following questions can evaluate the potential effects of ethnic minority status and transnational family ecologies on couple acculturation experiences:

- Have you ever been treated poorly in this country because of your race or ethnic heritage? How did you feel when you experienced this? How did you cope with this individually and as a couple? How has this experience affected your couple relationship?
- Before moving to the United States, what did you know about the ethnic groups who lived in this country? What have your interactions with other ethnic groups been like while living in the United States? Have these experiences influenced how you feel about living in this country?
- What is the ethnic composition of your neighborhood and city/town? Are there any Asian cultural organizations and social groups? How has this affected your ability to establish a new life together in this country?
- How often do you visit or contact family, friends, or business associates in your country of origin or other countries? What is the nature of these visits/contacts? Do you feel that these visits/contacts have helped you to adjust to this country as a couple? For example, do you feel that this has helped you to maintain certain cultural traditions or maintain your cultural identity in the United States?

Conclusion

Assessing family acculturation at the very outset of therapy not only helps to identify key acculturation issues and stressors that affect family functioning but it can also help clinicians adjust their therapeutic stance and treatment approach with Asian American families of variable acculturation levels. Immigrant families who possess different acculturation levels may have altogether different treatment expectations, illness and health conceptualizations, and therapy goals [60, 61]. By assessing how acculturation is manifested in a particular family across its different subsystems, clinicians can better understand how to join and work with family members within their culturally prescribed family structure and family roles. It is important to note, however, that although structural family therapy and family systems approaches provide helpful conceptual frameworks to comprehend the nature of family acculturation processes, their proscribed family therapy techniques may not necessarily be culturally appropriate for all Asian American families. This is especially the case for interventions calling for direct and open communication between family members, which can potentially violate traditional Asian American family role expectations and cultural norms regarding public expression of emotions and conflict. Clinicians also should be very clear about the purpose and nature of the recommended assessment questions presented in this chapter. Normalizing family acculturation difficulties and conflicts to diffuse associated loss of face concerns is an important component of this assessment process. In addition, clinicians should explain that individual interviews might be necessary to obtain a more complete picture of the whole family. Breaking up the family for separate interviews may increase their suspiciousness and ambivalence about therapy, but if this process is handled in a culturally appropriate manner, cultural misunderstandings can be minimized and certain family members may feel more comfortable speaking privately with the clinician [30, 49].

Lastly, although specific acculturation issues and patterns have been identified for different family subsystems, clinicians should avoid overgeneralizing these patterns to all Asian American families. Clinicians should not assume that all Asian American families are new immigrants to the United States and that all reported family problems, including parent–child and marital conflicts, are direct outcomes of acculturation. Almost thirty percent of Asian Americans are born in the United States and have lived in this country for multiple generations; thus acculturation conflicts and issues may not be their primary reasons for seeking therapy. At the same time, however, if an Asian American family has resided in the United States for an extensive period or multiple generations, clinicians should not assume that acculturation is irrelevant to their presenting problems. For example, Japanese Americans who have lived in the United States for several generations may actually be more traditional in certain ways than more recent Japanese immigrants because their cultural values reflect those of their grandparents who were raised in Japan at the beginning of the twentieth century [62]. Thus, certain Asian cultural values and traditions that are passed down to later generations may be "frozen" in time and become the basis for intergenerational family conflict. Lastly, clinicians should also be cautious about attributing family problems to acculturation when a more direct or alternative explanation is perhaps more logical. Conflict in Asian American families might simply reflect normative developmental family issues and changes – parent–child conflict might simply stem from an adolescent's desire to seek greater autonomy, and marital conflict might primarily reflect a new couple's struggles to negotiate the parameters and expectations of their young relationship. Nonetheless, all of these considerations are important reminders that Asian American families function and develop in complex ways, requiring new and more flexible family acculturation assessment approaches beyond individual self-report measures. The parent–child and couple assessment questions included in this chapter are intended to directly address this issue by allowing Asian American family members to share their acculturation experiences from their own perspectives in deeper and richer ways that potentially benefit therapy.

References

1. Nguyen NN, von Eye HH. The Acculturation Scale for Vietnamese Adolescents (ASVA): A bidimensional perspective. Int J Behav Assess 2002;26:202–213.
2. Ryder AG, Alden LE, Pauhus DL. Is acculturation unidimensional or bidimensional? A head-to-head comparison in the prediction of personality, self-identity, and adjustment. J Pers Soc Psych 2000;79:49–65.
3. Ward C, Kennedy A. Acculturation strategies, psychological adjustment, and sociocultural competence during cross-cultural transitions. Int J Intercult Rel 1994;18:329–343.
4. Chang T, Tracey TJG, Moore, TL. The dimensional structure of Asian American acculturation: An examination of prototypes. Self Identity 2005;4:25–43.
5. Kim BSK, Omizo MM. Asian and European American cultural values, collective self-esteem, acculturative stress, cognitive flexibility, and general self-efficacy among Asian American college students. J Couns Psychol 2005;52:412–419.
6. Chun KM, Eastman K, Wang G, Sue S. Psychopathology. In: Zane NWS, Lee L, eds. Handbook of Asian American psychology. Thousand Oaks, CA: Sage, 1998: 457–483.
7. Constantine MG, Okazaki S, Utsey SO. Self-concealment, social self-efficacy, acculturative stress, and depression in African, Asian, and Latin American International College Students. Am J Orthopsychiat 2004;74:230–241.
8. Mui AC, Kang SK. Acculturative stress and depression among Asian immigrant elders. Soc Work 2006;51:243–255.
9. Ying YW, Han M. The longitudinal effect of intergenerational gap in acculturation on conflict and mental health in Southeast Asian American adolescents. Am J Orthopsychiat 2007;77:61–66.
10. Balls Organista P, Organista KC, Kurasaki K. The relationship between acculturation and ethnic minority mental health. In: Chun KM, Organista PB, Marin G, eds. Acculturation: Advances in theory, measurement, and applied research. Washington, DC: American Psychological Association, 2003: 139–161.
11. Chun KM, Organista PB, Marin G, eds. Acculturation: Advances in theory, measurement, and applied research. Washington, DC: American Psychological Association, 2003.
12. Reeves T, Bennett C. The Asian and Pacific Islander population in the United States: March 2002, Current Population Reports, P20–P540. Washington, DC: US Census Bureau, 2003.
13. Hoffman L. Foundations of Family Therapy: A Conceptual Framework for Systems Change. New York, NY: Basic Books, 1981.
14. Chun KM. Conceptual and measurement issues in family acculturation research. In: Bornstein MH, Cote LR, eds. Acculturation and parent–child relationships: Measurement and development. Mahwah, NJ: Lawrence Erlbaum Associates, 2006:63–78.
15. Satir V. Conjoint family therapy: A guide to theory and technique. Palo Alto, CA: Science and Behavior Books, Inc., 1967.
16. Chun, KM. Understanding the nature and process of acculturation: preliminary findings from two community-based studies of Chinese Americans in San Francisco. In: 115th Annual Convention of the American Psychological Association. San Francisco, CA; August 2008.
17. Chun KM. Religious organizations in San Francisco Chinatown: Sites of acculturation and adaptation for Chinese immigrants. In: Lorentzen, LA, JL Gonzalez, Chun, KM, Do, HD, eds. On the corner of bliss and nirvana: The intersection of religion, politics, and identity in new migrant communities. Durham, NC: Duke University Press, 2009.
18. Sue DW, Sue D. Counseling the culturally diverse: Theory and practice. 4th ed. New York, NY: Wiley, 2003.

19. Minuchin S. Families and family therapy. Cambridge, MA: Harvard University Press, 1974.
20. Kawahara DM, Fu M. The psychology and mental health of Asian American women. In: Leong FTL, Inman AG, Ebreo A, Yang LH, Kinoshita L, Fu M, eds. Handbook of Asian American psychology. 2nd ed. Thousand Oaks, CA: Sage, 2007:181–196.
21. Suh SH. Too maternal and not womanly enough: Asian-American women's gender identity conflict. Women Ther 2007;30:35–50.
22. Minuchin S, Fishman HC. Family therapy techniques. Cambridge, MA: Harvard University Press, 1981.
23. Bronfenbrenner U. Ecology of the family as a context for human development: Research perspectives. Dev Psychol 1986;22:723–742.
24. Yee BWK, Huang LN, Lew A. Families: Life-span socialization in a cultural context. In: Zane NWS, Lee L, eds. Handbook of Asian American psychology. Thousand Oaks, CA: Sage, 1998:83–136.
25. Yee BWK, DeBaryshe BD, Yuen S, Kim SY, McCubbin HI. Asian American and Pacific Islander families: Resiliency and life-span socialization in a cultural context. In: Leong FTL, Inman AG, Ebreo A, Yang LH, Kinoshita L, Fu M, eds. Handbook of Asian American psychology. 2nd ed. Thousand Oaks, CA: Sage, 2007:69–86.
26. Chun KM, Akutsu PD. Acculturation among ethnic minority families. In: Chun KM, Organista PB, Marin G, eds. Acculturation: Advances in theory, measurement, and applied research. Washington, DC: American Psychological Association, 2003:95–119.
27. Kinoshita L, Hsu J. Assessment of Asian Americans: Fundamental issues and clinical applications. In: Leong FTL, Inman AG, Ebreo A, Yang LH, Kinoshita L, Fu M, eds. Handbook of Asian American psychology. 2nd ed. Thousand Oaks, CA: Sage, 2007:409–428.
28. Sue S, Zane N. The role of culture and cultural techniques in psychotherapy: A critique and reformulation. Am Psychol 1987;42:37–45.
29. Gibbs JT, Huang LN. Children of color: Psychological interventions with culturally diverse youth. San Francisco, CA: Jossey-Bass, 1998.
30. Lee E. Working with Asian Americans: A guide for clinicians. New York, NY: Guilford Press, 1997.
31. Fong TP. The contemporary Asian American experience. 3rd ed. Upper Saddle River, NJ: Pearson Prentice Hall, 2008.
32. Sodowsky GR, Kwan KK, Pannu R. Ethnic identity of Asians in the United States. In: Ponterotto JG, Casas JM, Suzuki LA, Alexander CM, eds. Handbook of multicultural counseling. Thousand Oaks, CA: Sage, 1995:123–154.
33. Rosenthal DA, Feldman SS. The nature and stability of ethnic identity in Chinese youth: Effects of length of residence in two cultural contexts. J Cross Cult Psychol 1992;23:214–227.
34. Phinney JS, Chivera V. Ethnic identity and self-esteem: An exploratory longitudinal study. J Adolescence 1992;15:271–281.
35. Chiu LH. Child-rearing attitudes of Chinese, Chinese-Americans, and Anglo American mothers. Int J Psychol 1987;22:409–419.
36. Inman AG, Howard EE, Beaumont RL, Walker JA. Cultural transmission: Influence of contextual factors in Asian Indian immigrant parents' experiences. J Couns Psychol 2007;54:93–100.
37. Kim H, Chung RHG. Relationship of recalled parenting style to self-perception in Korean American college students. J Genet Psych 2003;164:481–492.
38. Lin C, Fu VR. A comparison of child-rearing practices among Chinese, immigrant Chinese, and European-American parents. Child Dev 1990;61:429–433.
39. Nguyen L, Huang LN. Understanding Asian American youth development: A social ecological perspective. In: Leong FTL, Inman AG, Ebreo A, Yang LH, Kinoshita L, Fu

M, eds. Handbook of Asian American psychology. 2nd ed. Thousand Oaks, CA: Sage, 2007:87–103.
40. Tsai JL, Ying YW, Lee PA. The meaning of "being Chinese" and "being American": Variation among Chinese American young adults. J Cross Cult Psychol 2000;31: 302–332.
41. Kim BLC, Ryu E. Korean families. In: McGoldrick M, Giordano J, Garcia-Preto N. Ethnicity and family therapy. 3rd ed. New York, NY: Guilford Press, 2005:349–362.
42. McQuillan J, Tse, L. Child language brokering in linguistic minority communities: Effects on cultural interaction, cognition, and literacy. Lang Educ 1995;9:195–215.
43. Tse L. Language brokering in linguistic minority communities: The case of Chinese- and Vietnamese-American students. Biling Res J 1996;20:485–498.
44. Chao R. The prevalence and consequences of adolescents' language brokering for their immigrant parents. In: Bornstein MH, Cote LR, eds. Acculturation and parent-child relationships: Measurement and development. Mahwah, NJ: Lawrence Erlbaum, 2006: 271–296.
45. Wells M, Jones, R. Childhood parentification and shame-proneness: A preliminary study. Am J Fam Ther 2000;28:18–27.
46. Lopez GR. The value of hard work: Lessons on parent involvement from an immigrant household. Harvard Educ Rev 2001;71:416–437.
47. Orellana MF. The work kids do: Mexican and Central American immigrant children's contributions to households and schools in California. Harvard Educ Rev 2001;71:366–389.
48. Orellana MF. Responsibilities of children in Latino immigrant homes. In: Fuligni A, ed. New directions for youth development: Theory, practice and research, special issue on social influences in the positive development of immigrant youth. San Francisco, CA: Jossey-Bass, 2003:25–39.
49. McGoldrick M, Giordano J, Garcia-Preto N. Ethnicity and family therapy. 3rd ed. New York, NY: Guilford Press, 2005.
50. Chun, KM, Akutsu PD, Abueg FR. A study of Southeast Asian veterans of the Vietnam War. In: 28th Annual Convention of the Association for Advancement of Behavior Therapy, San Diego CA; November 1994.
51. Hall GCN. Culture-specific ecological models of Asian American violence. In: Hall GCN, Okazaki S, eds. Asian American psychology: The science of lives in context. Washington, DC: American Psychological Association, 2002:153–170.
52. Kim IJ, Lau AS, Chang DF. Family violence among Asian Americans. In: Leong FTL, Inman AG, Ebreo A, Yang LH, Kinoshita L, Fu M, eds. Handbook of Asian American psychology. 2nd ed. Thousand Oaks, CA: Sage, 2007:363–378.
53. Ho CK. An analysis of domestic violence in Asian American communities: A multicultural approach to counseling. Women Ther 1990;9:129–150.
54. Masaki B, Wong L. Domestic violence in the Asian community. In: Lee E, ed. Working with Asian Americans: A guide for clinicians. San Francisco, CA: Guilford Press, 1997:439–451.
55. Iwamasa GY, Sorocco KH. The psychology of Asian American older adults. In: Leong FTL, Inman AG, Ebreo A, Yang LH, Kinoshita L, Fu M, eds. Handbook of Asian American psychology. 2nd ed. Thousand Oaks, CA: Sage, 2007:213–226.
56. Kao, RSK, Lam ML. Asian American elderly. In: Lee E, ed. Working with Asian Americans: A guide for clinicians. San Francisco, CA: Guilford Press, 1997: 208–223.
57. Mui AC, Domanski MD. A community needs assessment among Asian American elders. J Cross Cult Gerontol 1999;14:77–90.
58. Mui AC, Nguyen DD, Kang D, Domanski MD. Demographic profiles of Asian immigrant elderly residing in metropolitan ethnic enclave communities. J Ethnic Cultur Divers Soc Work 2007;15:193–214.

59. Lorentzen, LA, JL Gonzalez, Chun, KM, Do, HD, eds. On the corner of bliss and nirvana: The intersection of religion, politics, and identity in new migrant communities. Durham, NC: Duke University Press, 2009.
60. Leong FTL, Chang, DF, Lee SH. Counseling and psychotherapy with Asian Americans: Process and outcomes. In: Leong FTL, Inman AG, Ebreo A, Yang LH, Kinoshita L, Fu M, eds. Handbook of Asian American psychology. 2nd ed. Thousand Oaks, CA: Sage, 2007:429–447.
61. Nagayama Hall GC, Eap S. Empirically supported therapies for Asian Americans. In: Leong FTL, Inman AG, Ebreo A, Yang LH, Kinoshita L, Fu M, eds. Handbook of Asian American psychology. 2nd ed. Thousand Oaks, CA: Sage, 2007:429–447.
62. Asai MO, Kameoka VA. The influence of Sekentei on family caregiving and underutilization of social services among Japanese caregivers. Soc Work 2005;50:111–118.

The A-B-C in Clinical Practice with Southeast Asians: Basic Understanding of Migration and Resettlement History

Khanh T. Dinh

Abstract This chapter focuses on the adjustment experiences of Southeast Asian (SE Asian) refugees and immigrants in the United States. Subtopics to be covered include the following: SE Asian populations in the United States, premigration and migration history, resettlement and adaptation in the United States, changes in SE Asian families and social network, mental health issues among SE Asians, and implications for clinical practice with SE Asians. This chapter highlights the importance of understanding premigration, migration, and resettlement issues in the provision of clinical services to SE Asian individuals and families.

Keywords Southeast Asian refugees and immigrants · Premigration and migration history · Resettlement and Adaptation · Southeast Asian American families · Southeast Asian American mental health · Clinical practice with Southeast Asian American families

Contents

SE Asian Populations in the United States	124
Premigration and Migration History	125
Resettlement and Adaptation in the United States	128
Changes in SE Asian Families and Social Network	132
Mental Health Issues among SE Asians	134
Implications for Clinical Practice with SE Asians	137
Conclusion	138
References	138

Specifically in the Asian community, Southeast Asians (SE Asians) represent one of the more recent refugee/immigrant populations in the United States. Clinical practice with SE Asians requires a basic knowledge of their

K.T. Dinh (✉)
University of Massachusetts Lowell, Department of Psychology, Lowell, MA, USA
e-mail: khanh_dinh@uml.edu

premigration, migration, and resettlement history, providing key contextual information for understanding their acculturative and adjustment experiences, especially their mental health issues. This chapter on SE Asians briefly covers the following topics: SE Asian populations in the United States, premigration and migration history, resettlement and adaptation in the United States, changes in SE Asian families and social network, mental health issues among SE Asians, and implications for clinical practice with SE Asians. Needless to say, this chapter does not represent an exhaustive discussion of SE Asians in the United States but only hopes to provide some basic knowledge of migration and resettlement history and some guidance in clinical practice with this population.

Why is it important to have a basic understanding of migration and resettlement history in clinical practice with SE Asians? For clinicians and mental health providers who regularly work with refugee and immigrant populations, the answer to this question is apparent, but it may not be the case for other clinicians. To demonstrate this point, a few years ago I received a phone call from a colleague needing some consultation help on a clinical case concerning a Vietnamese female client in her 30s. She had been providing treatment to her client for several months, who presented clinical symptoms of depression and suicidal ideation. My colleague was feeling somewhat stuck in her treatment provision and uncertain of the next therapeutic steps or assessment. I then asked my colleague what she could tell me about her client's immigrant background, whether she was born outside the United States, and if so, when had she immigrated to the United States, and her adjustment experiences to life in this country. Her response was unexpected – there was a brief pause and then she stated, "It did not occur to me to ask about her immigrant background." This example demonstrates the importance of having some basic knowledge of migration and resettlement history in clinical practice with SE Asians as it can help guide assessment and treatment design, and provide insights for understanding clients' experiences of acculturation and adaptation, family dynamics, and mental health symptoms.

SE Asian Populations in the United States

Who are the SE Asians? The region of SE Asia includes 11 different countries, but the term "SE Asian refugees" typically refers to people from Vietnam, Laos, or Cambodia. Another term that is often used to label these SE Asian people is "Indochinese," although this term is not preferable as a self-label and stems from past French colonialism in the region. There were few Vietnamese, Laotians, or Cambodians living in the United States prior to 1975 [1, 2] but now they can be found in every state in the United States, thus increasing the chances of mental health professionals coming into contact with SE Asian individuals and families.

Vietnamese, approximately 1,400,000 people, comprise the largest SE Asian refugee and immigrant group and currently represent the fourth largest

Asian American population in the United States [3]. California (539,000) and Texas (159,000) have the two largest Vietnamese populations, followed by Washington (61,000), Florida (56,000), Massachusetts (49,000), and Virginia (48,000). Orange County, California, is home to the largest concentration of Vietnamese outside of Vietnam (233,573) [4], with "Little Saigon" as its cultural and civic center.

Laotians, approximately 385,000 people, comprise the second largest SE Asian refugee and immigrant group in the United States [5]. Laotians include many different ethnic groups but the two largest groups are the Highland Hmong (183,000) and the Lowland Lao (193,000). California is home to the largest Hmong (65,000) and Lao (63,000) populations, but sizable communities of one or both of these two groups can also be found in Minnesota, Wisconsin, Texas, and Washington [3].

Cambodians, approximately 217,000 people, comprise the third largest SE Asian refugee and immigrant group in the United States [3]. California (84,000) is home to the largest Cambodian community in the United States, followed by Massachusetts (24,000) as the second largest community. Other sizable communities of Cambodians can be found in Washington (16,000), Texas (12,000), Florida (8,000), and Pennsylvania (6,000).

Premigration and Migration History

The Vietnam War is synonymous with SE Asian refugees in America because the end of this war in 1975, when American military power collapsed in the region, prompted the beginning of a lengthy mass exodus of Vietnamese, Laotian, and Cambodian refugees and immigrants. While the Vietnam War was centralized in Vietnam, this military conflict expanded into Laos and Cambodia, also devastating these neighboring countries and people [6]. Many fled from the region due to fears of persecution from the emerging communist governments in their respective countries.

The majority of SE Asian families and individuals confronted varying degrees of war-related trauma prior to their exodus from their countries. For example, large segments of the Vietnamese population were already refugees within their own country, as the Vietnam War (1959–1975) intensified and destroyed many regions of Vietnam, forcing them to flee from their homes. It was estimated that at least two million Vietnamese, of which many were civilians, died during the Vietnam War [6]. Furthermore, many Vietnamese adults and elders have had a long history of trauma from previous wars in Vietnam (Japanese invasion during World War II and French Indochina War), indicating multiple traumatic experiences in their lifetime (this is also the case for other SE Asian refugees). In my past clinical work with Vietnamese adults and elders at a refugee services agency, especially those who were originally from North Vietnam, many described war-related experiences associated with previous wars, such as witnessing the death, killing, and/or rape of family members and the difficulties of leaving their relatives in the North to flee to the South due to fears of persecution by the North Vietnamese communist government. Vietnamese who fought on the French side during the Indochina War or were part of the upper-class landowners faced persecution from the North Vietnamese communist government when France lost the war in 1954; Vietnam was partitioned into two countries, North Vietnam – Democratic Republic of Vietnam and South Vietnam – Republic of Vietnam [6].

In the case of Cambodian refugees, many witnessed the death or killing of loved ones and the destruction of their society and culture by Pol Pot and the Khmer Rouge, a communist government that controlled Cambodia from 1975 to 1979. They were the architect of the Cambodian genocide or "killing fields" that resulted in the deaths or killing of at least one million Cambodians [7]. According to a study published in the *Journal of the American Medical Association* [8], almost all (99%) of a Cambodian community sample from Long Beach, California, reported experiences of near-death starvation. In addition, 96% endured forced labor, 90% reported having a family member or friend murdered, 85% witnessed beatings, 56% witnessed killings, and 54% were tortured. An account by Arn Chorn-Pond, a survivor of the Cambodian genocide and an internationally recognized human rights activist and musician, depicts the horror experienced by many Cambodian individuals:

> I was in a temple where they killed three or four times a day. They told us to watch and not to show any emotion at all. They would kill us if we reacted... if we cried, or showed that we cared about the victims. They would kill you right away. So I had to shut it all off... I can shut off everything in my body, practically, physically. I saw them killing people right in front of me... The blood was there, but I didn't smell it. I made myself numb... The killing was unbearable. You go crazy if you smell the blood (9, p. 28).

In the case of Laotians, especially the Hmong, they were recruited by the US Central Intelligence Agency and worked closely with the US military to fight in an American "secret war" that was an extension of the Vietnam War. The main goal was countering communist forces in Laos and Vietnam. When the United States withdrew from Vietnam, the Hmong and other Laotians who sided with the US military became targets for persecution and genocide by the Pathet Lao, an insurgent group that established a Marxist government in Laos, with the support of the Vietnamese communist government [10]. It was estimated that about one-third of the Hmong population died during the war and many thousands more died in concentration/labor camps. Therefore, it is not unexpected that the majority of Hmong families in the United States had experienced the death or murder of family members and friends [11].

The exodus of refugees and immigrants from Vietnam, Laos, and Cambodia occurred through various waves and routes, whether by air, sea, or land. Many died or were killed in the process and many had to leave family members behind and/or were separated from family members during their escape from their home country. It is important to note that not all SE Asians living in the United States entered this country under refugee status, as defined by the US government, because a large segment of the population came to America through the family reunification program that is still in place today. This is not to say that the latter group does not have histories of trauma from the Vietnam War or persecution from their governments in their respective countries. The diverse premigration and migration experiences of SE Asians as well as their diverse backgrounds are important to keep in mind, in both research and clinical practice.

The Vietnamese exodus occurred in three major waves. The first wave of Vietnamese refugees, approximately 132,000 people, escaped Vietnam, via air and sea, immediately following the fall of Saigon (now renamed as Ho Chi Minh City) in April 1975 due to fears of persecution [12]. These refugees were generally better educated, wealthier, more familiar with the English language and Western cultures, and had some connections with the US government, military, or companies as compared with Vietnamese refugees or immigrants of subsequent waves. The second wave of refugees from Vietnam (1977–1982), about 400,000 people that included many Chinese-Vietnamese individuals and families, is often known as the "boat people" because the majority escaped from Vietnam onboard small, overcrowded fishing boats [1]. As a result, many individuals lost their lives at sea or were victims of robbery, rape, and/or murder by Thai pirates. Many had tales similar to this one, recounted by a Chinese-Vietnamese male refugee:

> Our boat had just departed for a short distance when another pirate boat attacked. The [boat] owner did not stop. They hit and destroyed the edge of one side of our boat. We were very scared. Not very long after, more pirate boats arrived and surrounded us. This time they could not find anything, so they wanted women and children to go to their boat. No one made a move. At the same time, they found gold hidden by the [boat] owner... They were satisfied. We were lucky. Because the pirates got gold, girls and women were not raped. After we arrived in camp we learned that those on almost every boat that arrived after us were raped and robbed... (13, pp. 31–32).

Those who escaped drowning, starvation, and/or victimization typically ended up in refugee camps in Thailand and other neighboring countries, where they spent months or even years before receiving permanent asylum in another country. The third wave of about 530,000 people included mostly immigrants, as opposed to refugees, who were allowed by the Vietnamese government to leave Vietnam (1982–present). They were given permission, through an agreement with the United Nations, to reunite with family members already living in the United States and other countries [14].

The largest exodus of refugees from Cambodia occurred in 1978–1979, when Vietnam invaded Cambodia and overthrew Pol Pot and the Khmer Rouge, as part of their response to a series of invasions into Vietnam by the Khmer Rouge [7]. During this extremely chaotic period (the Pol Pot overthrow coupled with the genocide and destruction of Cambodia since 1975), thousands of Cambodians fled to Thailand and other neighboring countries. Many died or were killed during their flight through jungles and landmines. Similar to the experiences of the second wave of refugees from Vietnam, Cambodians found themselves in refugee camps for months or years before permanent resettlement in another country. Life in the overcrowded refugee camps was far from ideal as camps were hastily put together by the United Nation High Commissioner for Refugees, with little provision of resources and basic needs. In addition, the camps were often attacked at night by the Khmer Rouge rebels who were hiding in the jungles from Vietnamese military forces. It has been speculated that there were many former Khmer Rouge members living among the refugees in these camps and subsequently resettled in the United States and elsewhere [7]. Of the hundreds of thousands of Cambodians in the refugee camps, only about 150,000 were allowed to resettle in the United States between 1975 and 1994, with most arriving in the early and mid-1980s.

The exodus of refugees from Laos, including the Highland Hmong and Lowland Lao, began in 1975 as thousands of people fled to Thailand to escape genocide, persecution, and re-education/concentration camps. Similar to the experiences of other SE Asian refugee groups, many individuals died or were killed during flight and those who survived and arrived in Thailand spent lengthy periods in refugee camps, under substandard conditions, prior to permanent resettlement in another country. A Hmong woman described her experiences in a refugee camp in Thailand:

> We would wait and wait for the next truck of food to arrive. It was almost impossible to survive on what we got. Each time the truck came, they had like a bowl, and they would measure one bowl per a family member. So if you have six people in your family, you will be given six bowls for two weeks. I mean – there is no way... I ate the food so preciously, not to waste a single rice grain. Most of the time I was still hungry, but I had to give up whatever I could to my children. It was so sad and so hard... In the camp we were in jail, like the chickens and pigs in Laos. We were that helpless and trapped. We ate only what we were given and when we were given, and if they didn't want to give us we would just starve (15, p. 71–72).

The circumstances of the Hmong were unique as they were recruited by the CIA to fight for the United States during the Vietnam War. In fact, when the United States lost the war in 1975, the Hmong thought that the US government would facilitate their safe exodus from Laos but this failed to materialize. The Hmong were left to fend for themselves against communist forces. Therefore, many still feel a sense of betrayal and mistrust of the US government. Because of this history, the US government, to some extent, felt obligated to receive refugees from Laos, especially the Hmong who fought for the US military. A few thousand refugees were allowed to come to the United States starting in late 1975, and by 1990, about 100,000 Hmong and Lao had resettled in the United States [16].

Resettlement and Adaptation in the United States

Difficulties and challenges did not magically disappear once SE Asian refugees found themselves safely in the United States, but instead were further compounded by the overwhelming stress associated with starting a new life in a new land. Although there were varying resettlement experiences across groups and within each group, there were also some common experiences. Unlike the experiences of Cuban refugees who were able to resettle within one central location in the United States, many SE Asian refugee individuals and families were systematically dispersed throughout the country, a policy implemented by the US government to discourage the formation of ethnic enclaves and to minimize the impact of refugee resettlement on any particular geographical area. Hence, many refugees found themselves in various cities and rural communities across the country with little or no access to other SE Asian refugees or to existing Asian American communities, posing additional challenges in their adjustment process in America. For example, Chan [7] highlights the resettlement experience of a Cambodian teenaged girl, recalled years later in adulthood, who, along with her family, was sponsored by a farm owner in Georgia that conveyed deep feelings of isolation and helplessness:

> When the sponsor took us away, she treated us as slaves. My Mom was working in their house, cleaning their house every day... We all worked like crazy. I had to go work in the fields and then come back to the house to work every day... washing their clothes, cleaning their house, things like that. And I got only $20 a week... My brother had problems, he went to the doctor and had operations many times. The thing that really pained me, that really hurt me, was that when he arrived home, the very next day they asked him when he could start working again. We were handicapped. We didn't know where to find help (p. 84).

Unfortunately, negative experiences with sponsors were not uncommon among SE Asian refugees; the stress endured during the initial resettlement subsequently can have long-term effects on adjustment and mental health issues [17].

Within a few years of the initial resettlement, what was observed was the beginning of a significant pattern of secondary migration toward regions with higher concentrations of SE Asians and/or other Asian Americans, namely to states such as California, Texas, Minnesota, Washington, and Massachusetts, creating sizable ethnic enclaves in various geographical areas. This was not unexpected and represented an appropriate coping reaction as ethnic enclaves do provide important resources and support for refugees and immigrants.

Another common resettlement experience among SE Asian refugees was that many were sponsored or assisted by religious organizations, such as the Migration and Refugee Services of US Catholic Conferences, Church World Service, Lutheran Immigration and Refugee Service, and the World Relief Refugee Services of the National Association of World Evangelicals. These organizations, often referred to as Voluntary Resettlement Agencies or VOLAGs, worked in tandem with federal, state, and local governments in the resettlement process. Although many religious sponsors were instrumental in helping SE Asian refugees adjust to their new life in America (e.g., assistance in housing, employment, and English language acquisition), some were more interested in converting the refugees to their religion [18], as demonstrated by the following experience of a Vietnamese refugee male:

> My sponsor asked me to go to his church, but I cannot go [because] I am Buddhist. I could not say "no" because I do not want to be ungrateful for all his help. So I say "yes"

> to make him feel good and know that I like him. When I did not go, he called and was upset, but he did not say why (14, p. 45).

Similar to the case above, many of the refugees felt a sense of obligation to attend church services and Bible study as a way to express their gratitude for the churches' generosity and help even though they did not share their sponsors' religious beliefs. This and other religious pressures certainly added another dimension of stress that further complicated the adjustment experiences of SE Asians.

Once resettled in the United States, SE Asian refugees soon realized the additional challenges of adjusting to American life. Most experienced cultural shock although the degree of severity partially depended on the characteristics of the refugees, such as their age, gender, premigration socioeconomic status, and level of education, and the extent to which they were exposed to American culture and language prior to emigration from their home country. These and other individual characteristics, along with contextual and historical factors, were influential during and beyond the initial resettlement period, and also impacted their on-going acculturative experiences. The following excerpt by a Hmong male demonstrates the impact of age on his adjustment to life in America:

> Life in America is very tough for me because I'm old. I'm sixty-five now and can't do anything. I would rather go back if I had the choice. I have been here so long, but I have not learned how to speak English or how to write. I tried but it was not easy... I guess as you get older, things just appear harder to learn... I am very frustrated. I thought by coming to America I would find a new life. I did – but it is harder than in Laos (15, p. 101).

The challenges of adapting to American life and society ranged from simple mundane matters, such as learning how to operate household appliances, grocery shopping, using American money, and navigating through public transportation systems, to more complex matters, such as learning a new language, adopting culturally appropriate behaviors and communication style, attending school, and searching for employment [19]. Many SE Asian refugees, especially those who were resettled in colder regions and away from the coasts, also had to adjust to drastic changes in geography and climate. Although there are numerous individual differences within each SE Asian refugee group, generally the Vietnamese, especially those of the first wave, fared somewhat better than the Cambodian, Laotians, and Hmong [20]. In all groups, those with higher levels of education and English proficiency, and those younger in age were in a relatively better position to cope with the cultural shock and acculturative process.

Another common resettlement experience was that the majority of SE Asian refugees started their new life in America on public assistance and at the bottom of the socioeconomic ladder. Many adult refugees began searching for employment soon after the initial resettlement with the main goal of establishing self-sufficiency and economic stability for their families. This was particularly important for adult male members, as employment represented a core aspect of male identity and respectability. As expected, considerable underemployment or unemployment was observed among many SE Asian adult males, requiring many adult females to attain work outside the home [21]. Economic challenges were and still remain a significant factor in the lives of SE Asians. According to data from the 1990 Census, 15 years after the initial arrival of SE Asian refugees to the United States, about 66% of Hmong/Laotian, 47% of Cambodian, and 34% of Vietnamese were living at or below the poverty level, well above the poverty rates of 10 and 14%, respectively, for the total US population and total Asian Pacific American population [22]. Ten years later, the 2000 Census indicated that 30% of Hmong, 22% of Cambodian, 14% of Laotians, and 10% of Vietnamese households were on public assistance. The rates of the Hmong and Cambodian were well above the national rate of 9.5%. These economic conditions suggest additional difficulties and challenges for SE Asians that, in turn, can impact other dimensions of adjustment and well-being.

The reception of SE Asian refugees by communities across America was initially positive, which was partly motivated by guilt associated with American involvement in the Vietnam War as well as genuine humanitarian concern for the welfare of the refugees. The initial positive reception, however, was not without some negative sentiments among host individuals and communities, perhaps partly due to some Americans still feeling bitter about American defeat in Vietnam, anti-Asian views during the 1970s and 1980s as a result of increasing Asian imports, a growing anti-immigrant attitude relating to native fears of losing jobs to immigrants, and/or misperceptions of SE Asian refugees as communists [23, 24]. There was also resentment of SE Asian refugees as welfare dependents. Unlike those of immigrant status, refugee status allowed SE Asian individuals and families immediate access to federal assistance programs, at least for the first 2 years of resettlement [25]. Because of this and other previously mentioned factors, as well as the continuing influx of SE Asian refugees into the country, by the late 1970s the majority of Americans surveyed in various Gallup polls preferred that SE Asian refugees be kept out of the United States [26]. While a great number of American individuals and communities, along with local, state, and federal governments, extended valuable assistance to SE Asian refugees, many of these refugees also confronted considerable resistance and discrimination in their adjustment process to American society. Many adult refugees faced discrimination during their search for employment and were victims of hate crimes [1], and many refugee youths faced discrimination within school settings:

> I was called "fish breath" and it made me angry. I am not a "chink" or a "slant eye." I do not like being called names and I know that most of my friends at school do not like it either [9th grade Vietnamese girl] (14, p. 95).

The systematic dispersion of refugees across the country and the lack of preexisting SE Asian communities most likely intensified the acculturative stress and challenges faced by SE Asian individuals and families. The different waves of SE Asian refugee and immigrant resettlement and the varied circumstances of their emigration from their home countries highlight numerous dimensions of diversity among SE Asians. SE Asians include those who have been in the United States for more than two decades as well as those who have just arrived; those who came with family members as well as those who came alone; and they all confronted varying degrees of difficulty and/or trauma in their departure from SE Asia and in their resettlement in America. Knowledge of migration and resettlement history provides a crucial backdrop for understanding the diverse life experiences of SE Asian individuals and families and their adaptation to American society.

Changes in SE Asian Families and Social Network

Migration and acculturative experiences can impact all aspects of life for SE Asian refugees and can have both short- and long-term effects. One area that is obvious is the impact on the family and social network. The change in cultural context has presented considerable challenges to many SE Asian families. These challenges are coupled with the fact that many refugees came to the United States with non-intact families. It is not uncommon to hear stories of a parent, a spouse, a sibling, and/or a child who were left behind in SE Asia, died during their departure or escape from the region, or were victims of genocide and war. For example, numerous Cambodian women are heads of household in single-parent families due to the deaths of their husbands or male family members during the Pol Pot era in Cambodia [27]. Therefore, the traumatic nature of premigration events and the exodus from their home countries has had a major impact on the size and make-up of many SE Asian families as well as the dynamics in family relationships. The traditional multigenerational pattern of kinship has been disrupted, which consequently leads to an incomplete system of family support and further intensifies the stress associated with the adjustment process to the American culture for many refugee families. Research of SE Asian young adults who have lived in the United States for an average of 11 years shows that those who have family members left behind in their country of origin reported a poorer quality of social support and family relationships (Dinh KT, Nemon M. The psychosocial profiles of immigrants in relation to migration and resettlement factors. Unpublished manuscript, 2007). Moreover, mental health problems of individual family members, especially those relating to past traumatic events, further complicate individual coping capacity and adjustment, which concurrently can affect the quality of family relationships and interactions [28].

As mentioned previously, changes in SE Asian families, especially in the dynamics of family relationships, family hierarchy and expectations, and gender roles, have been documented in the literature [24, 27, 29–31]. Relationships between family members, particularly between husband and wife and between parents and children, have been altered in significant ways as a result of confronting new cultural and economic demands as well as coping with the differential adaptation of individual family members. The changes in family relationships are partly due to changes in gender roles [28]. One aspect of the US culture that many SE Asian individuals have come to realize is the relatively more equal status between males and females, both within the US society and the mainstream American family. SE Asian men, who typically were the sole financial provider of their family in their home country, are no longer able to maintain that role in the United States as they find themselves underemployed or unemployed and on public assistance. The dramatic change in their social, occupational, and economic status serves to undermine the traditional male authority, especially the authority of the father or husband, in SE Asian families. This decrease in male authority is further affected by changes experienced by SE Asian females. Life in America, for the first time, affords many women/girls new opportunities, especially in the areas of employment and education. These new opportunities help women/girls to develop a degree of independence and identity separate from the prescribed traditional female roles, enabling them to realize their potential occupational skills and educational talents. While many SE Asian women have adjusted well to these changes in their lives, there are both positive and negative consequences. Many women experience a sense of accomplishment, especially in their ability to contribute to their family's financial welfare that goes beyond taking care of the household and children. On the other hand, they also feel overwhelmed by the changes in their roles, which entail work both outside and inside the home, as many SE Asian men hesitate in taking on domestic responsibilities that were traditionally defined as women's work. SE Asian men often feel threatened by the change in their wives' status and their own erosion of authority, which can create tension and conflict, sometimes leading to domestic violence, in spousal relations [25]. Although divorce is still highly stigmatized within SE Asian communities, this tension in the marital relationship perhaps partly explains the increase in divorce rates among SE Asians in America [7, 14].

Also as mentioned previously, another significant change in the traditional SE Asian family centers on parent–child relationships. The process of adaptation and acculturation to American culture typically differs between parents and children, which can lead to intergenerational conflicts [20]. The general pattern suggests that parents usually want to maintain core aspects of traditional culture and family values while their children tend to adopt more mainstream American values and lifestyles [32]. This differential pattern in adaptation is certainly influenced by differences in age and developmental stages of parents and children at the time of their arrival to the United States. Furthermore, parents and children are exposed to different socializing institutions (i.e., occupational/public assistance contexts for parents vs. school/peer contexts for children) that involve varying cultural and behavioral demands as suggested by the following excerpt from a Cambodian adult female recalling her high school experiences:

> My high school years mark the greatest achievement in terms of education but the greatest loss in terms of maintaining my own history, culture, and language. Like most teenagers, I wanted to be like everyone else... I wanted to assimilate into American society... The first thing I needed to do was to get rid of my Asian accent... I needed to

sound like an American whenever I opened my mouth. I was so determined to do this that I avoided speaking Khmer at all times. If my Mom spoke to me in Khmer, I answered her in English... I tried to distance myself from all aspects of Cambodian culture and history. Being normal meant having a background similar to that of my White American counterparts... It must have been hard for [my Mom] to watch me go through this process of disowning everything she had risked so much to teach me during the Khmer Rouge years (7, p. 213).

Within the school context, children learn from teachers and peers the importance of certain American values, such as individuality, independence, self-directedness, assertiveness, and questioning of authority. While incorporating these characteristics into their psychological and behavioral repertoire can facilitate educational success for children, the transfer of these characteristics into the SE Asian family context can lead to intergenerational problems and challenge the traditional roles and hierarchy of parents and children. Children may begin to question parental authority and other core aspects of filial piety, and their parents may believe that they are not accorded the respect and obedience they deserve. The parents' traditionally prescribed dominant roles within the family may be further lessened by their need to rely on their children's more proficient English language skills to cope with the demands and interactions of daily life in America [33, 34]. This is demonstrated by the following excerpt shared by a Vietnamese parent: "My son speaks English better [than me] and he does not speak Vietnamese good. Sometimes I have to get him for understanding [translating] and this I don't like. It makes him think he is better [than me]" (14, p. 127).

Changes in the parent–child relationships also may have different dynamics for sons and daughters [32]. Sons, especially the eldest one, may question the traditional obligations of sharing the same household with their parents and providing financial support and care for their aging parents, whereas daughters may question traditional gender roles in which females receive less opportunities and privileges than do their male siblings. These and other factors may negatively impact the overall quality of parent–child relationships in SE Asian families [35].

Compounding the complexities of parent–child relationships, many SE Asian parents and children have been so traumatized by war and migration experiences that neither party is in the best position to cope with and resolve intergenerational conflicts [20]. Often, these mental health problems (e.g., posttraumatic stress disorder (PTSD), depression, and anxiety) go untreated, which further perpetuate long-term difficulties for parents and children and further undermine the family network as the primary source of emotional and social support for all family members, especially for children [36, 37].

Mental Health Issues among SE Asians

The term "refugee" may indicate possible exposure to trauma, which consequently can impact the psychological adjustment of refugee individuals. SE Asian refugees confronted various traumatic events, such as the sudden and chaotic nature of departure and escape from their home country, separation or loss of family members during flight, rape and violence by pirates at sea, and/or years of horrendous living conditions in refugee camps. In thinking about these traumatic experiences, it is also important to consider the premigration trauma relating to war experiences. Prior to their exodus, many SE Asian refugees were also themselves refugees within their own country, as the Vietnam War and its related "secret wars" raged on and devastated many regions of Vietnam, Cambodia, and Laos. Many were also victims of persecution and labor camps and witnesses to violence and genocide. Thus, SE Asian refugees are at risk for developing mental health disorders, but experiences of trauma do not necessarily lead to mental health disorders. Other variables, such as personal coping capacity and resources, family network and support, English language proficiency, educational level, age, gender, along with other important historical, contextual, and resettlement variables, may serve as protective or risk factors in the development of mental health problems [38, 39].

It has been observed that mental health problems among SE Asian refugees, when they do begin to emerge, often occur within the initial period of 6–24 months after arriving in the United States [2, 14]. This suggests a delayed response to the refugee experience; only once refugees are safe and settled in their new environment and have time to reflect upon the dramatic changes and losses do mental health problems begin to emerge for individuals and families. One of the challenges in identifying mental health problems involves their meaning to SE Asian refugees. The term "mental health problem" or "mental illness or disorder" as defined in the United States is a foreign concept to many individuals, especially among those with less formal education and exposure to Western ideas and culture. In SE Asia, if a person is viewed as having a "mental illness," it means that he or she is "crazy" or has been invaded by spiritual entities and should be confined to the home or isolated from society. It also means that the person's family or ancestors must have committed some past misdeeds that now explain the current suffering of their family members or descendants. Therefore, individuals and families often endure mental health suffering while keeping their problems to themselves or within the family so as to avoid shame and guilt being placed on the family. In addition, as mentioned previously, another challenge in identifying mental health problems is the tendency for SE Asian individuals to express symptoms in somatic terms or bodily dysfunction [40]. This is a more acceptable way of conveying mental suffering that allows the person to receive some kind of medical treatment, even though it does not directly address the underlying psychological or psychiatric issues.

Despite these challenges, a number of mental health-related problems have been identified within SE Asian communities. Common examples include issues relating to traumatic experiences before and during their flight from their home country, issues relating to refugee camp conditions and length of stay, anxiety and fear associated with resettlement, homesickness, loneliness and isolation – especially for the elderly, poverty and loss of social status, loss of cultural values, stress associated with role changes, intergenerational conflicts, and unrealistic expectations among many refugees/immigrants about how good life would be in the United States [14, 20, 39]. These problems often are associated with symptoms of depression, suicidal ideation, anxiety, PTSD, alcohol abuse, and/or domestic violence [41–45].

One of the earlier studies on mental health issues of SE Asian refugees found that 71% were diagnosed with PTSD and 81% with depression [43]. Another study showed 50% suffered from PTSD and 71% from mixed anxiety and depression [45]. These studies, involving clinical samples, suggest high rates of mental illness among SE Asian refugee populations. Even with nonclinical samples, one study reported 36% with depression, 96% with anxiety, and 16% with PTSD [46], also indicating high rates of mental illness. It has been observed that among the different SE Asian subgroups, Cambodian and Hmong refugees exhibit the highest rates of mental health problems [47, 48], pointing to the importance of intergroup differences. One study involving a Cambodian sample found that 88% met the clinical criteria for anxiety, 86% for PTSD, and 80% for depression [49]. Differences within groups are also important to consider in clinical work with SE Asians. For example, among Vietnamese individuals, those from the second wave of refugee exodus reported more psychological distress than those from the first wave [38]. Other within-group differences, such as age, gender, English proficiency, and so on, should also be considered in clinical work with SE Asian populations. For example, mental health problems are more prevalent among SE Asian adults as compared with children or adolescents, and generally, adults experience more difficulties than do children in their transition to a new culture. Nonetheless, children may also suffer from adjustment and mental health problems, including those relating to exposure to trauma. Typically, these problems are associated with intergenerational conflicts, the challenges in navigating between their family culture and mainstream American culture, school adjustment, peer acceptance, and identity development [20, 24, 30]. Some commonly reported symptoms among SE Asian youths include depression, hopelessness, loneliness, anxiety, and low self-esteem [50–52].

While it is commonly believed that mental health problems among SE Asian refugee populations improve and eventually dissipate with time in the United States [33, 41], more recent research indicates a more complex pattern. In fact, it appears that traumatic events experienced before, during, and after migration can still have a major impact on the adjustment and mental health of many SE Asians, even 10 or 20 years later after resettlement in the United States. Nicholson [17], in a nonclinical sample of SE Asians with an average US residency of almost 10 years, found past traumatic experiences to be primary predictors of an individual's coping capacity of current life stressors, which, in turn, strongly predict current mental health problems. She also found that within her sample, 40% suffer from depression, 35% from anxiety, and 14% from PTSD. Marshall and colleagues [8], in their study of a community sample of 490 Cambodians who have been in the United States for more than 20 years, found high rates of PTSD (62%) and depression (51%), which were predicted by previous traumatic events experienced before and after migration. These more recent studies suggest the importance of attending to premigration, migration, and postmigration factors, even though they occurred more than two decades ago, in our conceptualization and understanding of SE Asians' current mental health issues and in our provision of clinical services. These studies also suggest the need for more long-term research, rather than just short-term within 3–5 years after resettlement, to provide a fuller temporal picture of refugee adjustment and adaptation.

Implications for Clinical Practice with SE Asians

When working with SE Asian clients, we must consider what types of questions should be included in our clinical assessment. As suggested throughout this chapter, a thorough assessment of premigration, migration, and resettlement experiences is crucial in establishing a basic foundation for understanding SE Asian clients' mental health problems and for treatment development.

With regard to *premigration* experiences, we should assess for demographic background, such as clients' level of education, socioeconomic status, and type of employment prior to migration. We certainly should ascertain their family background and history, including family composition and structure and what family life was like in their home country. This information can provide insights for understanding their current family situation. Information about their level of familiarity with American culture and language prior to migration is also helpful in understanding acculturation and adjustment issues. Of course, an assessment of premigration war and trauma exposure can help contextualize current presenting symptoms and difficulties, as well as their level of coping capacity and resilience.

Questions pertaining to SE Asian clients' *migration* or escape process are also important to assess in clinical settings. Examples of questions may include the following: Why did they decide to leave their home country, how was that decision made and who made that decision? Was the plan to leave well-thought out or was it a sudden decision to leave? Which family members were able to leave and who were left behind? What were the circumstances at the time of their departure from their home country? Were they confronted with difficulties and/or trauma during their migration or escape? These types of questions can inform us about the circumstances of their migration experiences and the way in which they coped with various challenges and trauma.

As stated previously, many SE Asians spent months or even years in refugee camps and so it is necessary to ascertain experiences pertaining to refugee camp living. Where was the location of the refugee camp – in which country? What was life like in the refugee camp? What about the living conditions and standards? What about hardships or difficulties that were confronted in the refugee camp? And how long were they living in the refugee camp? These questions further enhance our knowledge base of their life events and our understanding of their subsequent adjustment in the United States.

Finally, asking questions about SE Asian clients' *resettlement* experiences is also an important component of clinical assessment. Examples of questions include the location of their initial resettlement as well as secondary migration and reasons for their decision to relocate to another area. Who were their sponsors and the nature of their relationship with sponsors? What types of support and assistance did they receive from their sponsors? What attitudes and expectations did they have about life in the United States? What kinds of difficulties and challenges did they confront in resettlement, whether they were related to simple matters or complex ones? Did they experience discrimination, hate, or violence from host individuals or communities? In clinical practice, we often focus more on symptoms and negative events, but it is also important to assess for what they perceive as successes and achievements in their new life in America; while many SE Asian refugees and immigrants have confronted considerable hardships and trauma and are at higher risks for various mental health problems, they are strong survivors who have overcome much adversity.

Conclusion

In thinking about mental health issues among SE Asian refugees and immigrants, it is important to attend to migration and resettlement histories, as well as to key demographic, contextual, and environmental factors that may play influential roles in the manifestation of current mental health problems. This is necessary in our understanding of their life circumstances and presenting symptoms, and, of course, in our development and provision of clinical services that can effectively address the diverse mental health needs of SE Asians in America.

References

1. Takaki R. Strangers from a Different Shore: A History of Asian Americans. New York: Penguin Books, 1989.
2. Rumbaut RG. Vietnamese, Laotian, and Cambodian Americans. In: Min PG, ed. Asian Americans: Contemporary Trends and Issues. Thousand Oaks, CA: Sage Publications, 1995:232–270.
3. United States Census Bureau. American Fact Finder. Retrieved on 2 May 2007, from http://factfinder.census.gov, 2006.
4. United States Census Bureau. American Fact Finder. Retrieved on 2 November 2004, from http://factfinder.census.gov, 2000.
5. Southeast Asia Resource Action Center. Southeast Asian American Populations. Retrieved on 1 June 2007, from http://www.searac.org/poptable.html, 2007.

6. Karnow S. Vietnam: A History. New York: Penguin Books, 1997.
7. Chan S. Survivors: Cambodian Refugees in the United States. Urbana, IL: University of Illinois Press, 2004.
8. Marshall GN, Schell TL, Elliott MN, Berthold SM, Chun C. Mental health of Cambodian refugees 2 decades after resettlement in the United States. Journal of the American Medical Association 2005;294:571–579.
9. Simms L, Chorn-Pond A. Between tigers and crocodiles: An interview with Arn Chorn-Pond. Parabola: Myth, Tradition, and the Search for Meaning 2002;24:24–31.
10. Quincy K. Hmong: A History of a People. Spokane, WA: Eastern Washington University Press, 1995.
11. Tatman AW. Hmong history, culture, and acculturation: Implications for counseling the Hmong. Journal of Multicultural Counseling Psychology 2004;32:222–233.
12. Montero D. Vietnamese Americans: Patterns of Resettlement and Socioeconomic Adaptation in the United States. Boulder, CO: Westview Press, 1979.
13. Caplan N, Choy MH, Whitmore JK. Children of the Boat People: A Study of Educational Success. Ann Arbor, MI: The University of Michigan Press, 1991.
14. Rutledge PJ. The Vietnamese Experience in America. Bloomington, IN: Indiana University Press, 1992.
15. Faderman L, Xiong G. The Hmong and the American Immigrant Experience: I Begin My Life All Over. Boston, MA: Beacon Press, 1998.
16. Chan S. Hmong Means Free: Life in Laos and America. Philadelphia, PA: Temple University Press, 1994.
17. Nicholson B. The influence of pre-migration and post-migration stressors on mental health: A study of Southeast Asian refugees. Social Work Research 1997;21:19–31.
18. Beiser M, Turner J, Ganesan S. Catastrophic stress and factors affecting its consequences among Southeast Asian refugees. Social Science and Medicine 1989;28:183–195.
19. Uba L, Chung RC. The relationship between trauma and financial and physical well-being among Cambodians in the United States. The Journal of General Psychology 1991;118:215–225.
20. Uba L. Asian Americans: Personality Patterns, Identity, and Mental Health. New York: The Guilford Press, 1994.
21. Kibria N. Power, patriarchy, and gender conflict in the Vietnamese immigrant community. Gender and Society 1990;4:9–24.
22. Southeast Asia Resource Action Center. Economic and Professional Success Demographics. Retrieved on1 June 2007, from http://www.searac.org/statstab.html, 2007.
23. Starr P, Roberts A. Attitudes toward new Americans: Perceptions of Indo-Chinese in nine cities. Research in Race and Ethnic Relations 1982;3:165–186.
24. Zhou M, Bankston CL. Growing up American: How Vietnamese Children Adapt to Life in the United States. New York: Russell Sage Foundation, 1998.
25. Kibria N. Family Tightrope: The Changing Lives of Vietnamese Americans. Princeton, NJ: Princeton University Press, 1993.
26. Stern LM. Responses to Vietnamese refugees. Social Work 1981;26:306–311.
27. Boehnlein JK, Leung PK, Kinzie JD. Cambodian American families. In: Lee E, ed. Working with Asian Americans: A Guide for Clinicians. New York: The Guilford Press, 1997:37–45.
28. Chung RC, Bemak F. Revisiting the California Southeast Asian mental health needs assessment data: An examination of refugee ethnic and gender differences. Journal of Counseling and Development 2002;80:111–119.
29. Moore LJ, Keopraseuth K, Leung PK, Chao LH. Laotian American families. In: Lee E, ed. Working with Asian Americans: A Guide for Clinicians. New York: The Guilford Press, 1997:136–152.
30. Su J, Lee RM, Vang S. Intergenerational family conflict and coping among Hmong American college students. Journal of Counseling Psychology 2005;52:482–489.

31. Xiong ZB, Eliason PA, Detzner DF, Cleveland MJ. Southeast Asian immigrants' perceptions of good adolescents and good parents. The Journal of Psychology 2005;139:159–175.
32. Dinh KT, Sarason BR, Sarason IG. Parent–child relationships in Vietnamese immigrant families. Journal of Family Psychology 1994;8:471–488.
33. Rumbaut RG. The agony of exile: A study of the migration and adaptation of Indochinese refugee adults and children. In: Ahearn FL, Athley JL, eds. Refugee Children: Theory, Research and Services. Baltimore, MD: Johns Hopkins University Press, 1991:53–91.
34. Zhou M. Straddling different worlds: The acculturation of Vietnamese refugee children. In: Rumbaut RG, Portes A, eds. Ethnicities: Children of Immigrants in America. Berkeley, CA: University of California Press, 2001:187–227.
35. Dinh KT, Nguyen HH. The effects of acculturative variables on Asian American parent-child relationships. Journal of Social and Personal Relationships 2006;23:407–426.
36. Kinzie JD, Sack W. Severely traumatized Cambodian children: Research findings and clinical implications. In: Ahearn FL, Athley JL, eds. Refugee Children: Theory, Research and Services. Baltimore, MD: Johns Hopkins University Press, 1991:92–105.
37. Lam BT. An integrative model for the study of psychological distress in Vietnamese-American adolescents. North American Journal of Psychology 2005;7:89–106.
38. Chung RC, Bemak F, Wong S. Vietnamese refugees' levels of distress, social support, and acculturation: Implications for mental health counseling. Journal of Mental Health Counseling 2000;22:150–161.
39. Tran TV. Psychological traumas and depression in a sample of Vietnamese people in the United States. Health & Social Work 1993;18:184–194.
40. Kinzie JD. The establishment of outpatient mental health services for Southeast Asian refugees. In: Williams CL, Westermeyer J, eds. Refugee Mental Health in Resettlement Countries. New York: Hemisphere Publishing Corporation, 1986:217–231.
41. Beiser M. Influences of time, ethnicity, and attachment on depression in Southeast Asian refugees. American Journal of Psychiatry 1988;145:46–51.
42. Flaskerud JH, Nguyen AT. Mental health needs of Vietnamese refugees. Hospital and Community Psychiatry 1988;39:435–437.
43. Kinzie JD, Boehnlein JK, Leung PK, Moore LJ, Riley C, Smith D. The prevalence of posttraumatic stress disorder and its clinical significance among Southeast Asian refugees. American Journal of Psychiatry 1990;147:913–917.
44. Hinton WL, Chen Y-CJ, Du N, Tran CG, Lu FG, Miranda J, Faust S. DSM-III-R disorders in Vietnamese refugees: Prevalence and correlates. The Journal of Nervous and Mental Disease 1993;181:113–122.
45. Mollica RE, Wyshak G, Lavelle J. The psychiatric impact of war trauma and torture on Southeast Asian refugees. American Journal of Psychiatry 1987;144:1567–1572.
46. Gong-Guy E. The California Southeast Asian Needs Assessment. Oakland, CA: Asian Community Mental Health Services, 1986.
47. Molicca RE, Wyshak G, Lavelle J, Truong T, Tor S, Yang T. Assessing symptom change in Southeast Asian refugee survivors of mass violence and torture. American Journal of Psychiatry 1990;147:83–88.
48. Rumbaut RG. Mental health and the refugee experience: A comparative study of Southeast Asian refugees. In: Owan T, ed. Southeast Asian Mental Health: Treatment, Prevention, Services, Training, and Research. Washington, DC: US Department of Health and Human Services, 1985:433–456.
49. Carlson E, Rosser-Hogan E. Mental health status of Cambodian refugees ten years after leaving their homes. American Journal of Orthopsychiatry 1993;63:223–231.
50. Felsman JK, Leong FT, Johnson MC, Felsman IC. Estimates of psychological distress among Vietnamese refugees: adolescents, unaccompanied minors and young adults. Social Science Medicine 1990;31:1251–1256.

51. Fry PS. Stress ideations of Vietnamese youth in North America. The Journal of Social Psychology 1985;125:35–43.
52. Supple AJ, Small SA. The influence of parental support, knowledge, and authoritative parenting on Hmong and European American adolescent development. Journal of Family Issues 2006;27:1214–1232.

Clinical Considerations When Working with Asian American Children and Adolescents

Yanni Rho and Kathy Rho

Abstract There are a number of reasons Asian American children and adolescents are coming to the attention of mental health providers. In addition to the challenge of satisfactorily navigating through developmental stages, they may have to do so in a country whose culture and customs are either unfamiliar to their parents or to themselves. Other etiological reasons may include difficulties in identity formation and consolidation, including the compounded difficulties of simultaneous ethnic/sexual identity formation, acculturation challenges (e.g., acculturation gap between parents and children), and parental psychopathology, which can be challenging considering that many Asian parents may not recognize or seek help for themselves. Despite past research which has found Asian children and adolescents to have low rates of mental illness, there is also great evidence to support that illnesses and dysfunction such as depression, anxiety, suicidal ideation, substance abuse and dependence, and delinquent behaviors exist at significant rates and are critical concerns. This chapter will describe several points to consider when working with Asian children and their families in addition to special consideration for strength-based treatments when working with Asian American families. Finally, this chapter will conclude with a section providing clinical recommendations or considerations that may help provide the reader with a "frame" when working with acculturation stressors and their impact in Asian children and adolescents.

Keywords Asian American children and adolescents · Acculturation stressors · Intergenerational gap · Psychopathology in Asian American children and adolescents · Identity formation · Resiliency · Clinical recommendations with Asian children and adolescents

Y. Rho (✉)
Family, Youth, and Children's Services and Adult Services, Mental Health Division at the City of Berkeley; and private practice. Berkeley, CA, USA
e-mail: yrho@ci.berkeley.ca.us

Contents

For Children: Introduction to Clinical Considerations	145
For Adolescents: Introduction to Clinical Considerations	146
The Challenge of Identity Formation in Adolescence	147
Importance of Acculturation Assessment	148
Acculturation Gap: The Role of Children	148
Acculturation Gap: The Role of Parents	149
Parental Psychopathology and Impact on Children	149
Psychopathology in Asian Children and Adolescents	151
Somatized Distress	151
Depression	151
Anxiety	152
Suicide	153
Substance Abuse	154
Externalized Behaviors: Delinquency and Gang-Related Activity	155
Special Mention of Interethnic Dating and Gender/Sexuality Issues	156
Risk Factors and Resiliency	158
How do Children and Adolescents Come to Our Attention and What to Consider in Evaluation and Treatment	159
Clinical Considerations When Working with Children and Adolescents: General Thoughts	159
Work with Adolescents	161
Conclusion	162
References	163

Childhood is not simple and straightforward. There is the continual challenge of growth and development and the attainment of appropriate milestones in physical, emotional, cognitive, and social development. The children and adolescents of immigrants or those who are immigrants themselves may have additional challenges in development, for example, in identity consolidation. According to Erickson, throughout the life cycle, all humans are attempting to master different tasks. Childhood and adolescence, therefore, can be seen in terms of developmental stages. For the 3- to 6-year old, the challenge is to learn how to assert oneself and become more independent from parents and guardians ("initiative vs. guilt"). For the 6- to 12-year old, the task involves learning to incorporate and master many new skills ("industry vs. inferiority"). And finally, for the 12- to 18-year old, the challenge is to figure out who one is ("identity vs. role confusion") [1]. These tasks and stages can be challenging for children, adolescents, and their families. But for immigrant families, there may be a decreased ability for parents, friends, or teachers to help depending on factors such as difficulties in communication, emotional reserves and time available, and lack of understanding differences between culture of origin and new host culture.

This chapter addresses several aspects of development for Asian American children, adolescents, and their families, the conflicting reports and research that exist for Asian immigrant children and adolescents, the mental health of Asian American children and their families, and how to approach them clinically.

The authors are fully aware that although some generalizations may be made, it is vital to consider every child, adolescent, and their family as unique.

For Children: Introduction to Clinical Considerations

As mentioned previously, young children have the developmental task of trying to negotiate their world and learn new skills. At times, parents may be less equipped to help their children navigate through these developmental stages. In the families of immigrants, parents may not be able to help their children negotiate their new worlds due to language barriers and cultural unfamiliarity. This is compounded by the fact that children may learn English faster than their parents, incorporate their host country's cultural values and behaviors before their parents, and thus be expected to help their parents navigate life in their new country (e.g., America). Owing to these difficulties and others that will be further discussed in this chapter, it is not uncommon that Asian American children may struggle and require the assistance of mental health clinicians.

Clinically, children may come to our attention because of internalized reasons (when distress is manifest more inwardly such as depression or anxiety) or more externalized reasons (when distress is manifest more outwardly such as disruptive behaviors), especially if they are being referred by schools or for "abnormal" behaviors. To successfully engage a child and his/her family and perform a culturally sensitive evaluation, the impact of acculturation needs to be included in the assessment. For example, parents may have culturally sanctioned expectations for their children's behaviors; there may be a hesitance on the parents' part to disclose elements of their child's behavior, or there may be a misunderstanding and/or a lack of understanding about why the child was referred to seek help (e.g., if the child was referred by the pediatrician or by the school). And because many children may have limited understanding of these issues themselves, this may compound the clinician's ability to obtain an accurate history, identify the precise nature of the problem (whether internal or external), and ultimately, successfully work with children and their families on why and how the child is struggling.

Additional reasons that parents or schools might seek the help of a mental health clinician may be contingent on age or developmental stage of the child. For very young children, the referral may be made because the child is not achieving developmental milestones appropriately. Other reasons include concerns about language acquisition, difficulties adapting to school environments, poor performance in academics, and difficulties in behavior and willfulness. Regardless of the reason, it is important to consider that a culturally and linguistically sensitive evaluation must be performed for an accurate assessment. For example, this might include the use of culturally sensitive toys especially if the child is a recent immigrant (e.g., chopsticks vs. a fork if appropriate) for play therapy and assessment [2]. It is also important to get a sense of parental expectations of the child as well as school/other expectations of the child to obtain a good sense of why the child was referred. As stated previously, there are some behaviors that may be well tolerated at home but not well tolerated in a school setting and vice versa. For example, the school may not tolerate a child's tantrums, whereas they may be better tolerated at home due to a certain amount of permissiveness. Another example is a child who is assertive in school and is rewarded, but when assertive at home, they may be seen as the "bad" child.

Children and families may also be referred because child protection agencies may be alerted to and concerned about corporal punishment being used at home. Corporal punishment is commonly used in some Asian countries, for example, Korea [3], although it is well known to most that in America, it is not acceptable. It is especially important to be culturally sensitive, non-shaming, and provide communication that is judgment-free when providing education and guidance in the area of discipline. For example, one can inquire about how parents discipline their children in their home country and whether they are aware of how parents discipline in the United States. They can normalize the difficulties that come with the experience of trying to adapt to their new host culture including the method of disciplining (e.g., "time out" vs. spanking). In a similar manner, it is appropriate to educate the organizations that provide the referrals about the family that one works with and to correct misattributions, for example, bruising left by coining and cupping, which are folk remedies[1].

For Adolescents: Introduction to Clinical Considerations

There are several reasons that an Asian American adolescent may come to the attention of a mental health clinician. Depression and anxiety are of particular concern among Asian American adolescents, given that they may suffer quietly and neither be identified by others nor seek help for themselves. Negotiating the "identity vs. role confusion" stage is a particularly cumbersome challenge with multiple choice points, especially given the asymmetric acculturative process between themselves and their parents and the resultant role reversal [4]. Particularly in immigrant families, Asian American adolescents try to strike the balance between their role as "child" and "caregiver" and between Confucian/collective thinking and more independent, Westernized thinking, for example. This conflict is often intensified when traditional gender roles and expectations augment the responsibility and "obligation" of some adolescents to take care of their family and possibly other family members back in their home country [5].

---

[1] "Coining" refers to the folk remedy that entails running a coin along the body with herbal oils; "cupping" refers to the folk remedy that entails the use of suction cups that are to extract "bad winds" from the body.

Thus, Asian American adolescents in this situation are trying to consolidate their identities in the midst of many dilemmas, which may lead to both internalized and externalized difficulties.

The Challenge of Identity Formation in Adolescence

There are many different aspects of identity that one can possess and that one has to negotiate and master through development, especially during adolescence and young adulthood. More specifically, there are aspects of identity such as sexual identity (which will be addressed later in this chapter), gender identity, and ethnic/racial identity (which may be particularly challenging for immigrants as well as for biracial and adopted Asian children/adolescents). Erikson noted that identity forms in a sociocultural context. This context for children and adolescents usually consists of their larger community, schools, peers, and most importantly, families. This is particularly crucial in considering the determinants of identity formation in one's ethnic identity. Families can be an especially complicated factor in identity formation depending on how acculturated the parents are, how much the child or adolescent values parental expectations and beliefs, and how much conflict exists between parents and children. Ethnic identity (how one identifies or with which group they identify with most) is one aspect of identity in which the family can have enormous influence. For example, if a child's parents are very ethnically identified and the child has little conflict with their parents, the child may also be very ethnically identified. But if a child has great conflict with their parents, they may reject the ethnic part of their identity, possibly leading to further internal and external conflict.

Ego identity [1] can be discussed in terms of [1] whether someone has explored different identity options and [2] whether they have made a decision of which identity option to choose. The ego identity model proposes that there are four stages of ego identity development: diffuse (no exploration, no commitment), foreclosed (no exploration, commitment), moratorium (exploration, no commitment), and achieved (exploration, then commitment) [6]. *Exploration* refers to how much someone has investigated their identity options; *commitment* is whether or not someone has committed to certain aspects of their personality or ego identity. It has been found by previous authors that strong identity status correlates to higher self-esteem [7, 8]. But it is also noted that social context contributes to what stage an individual will move toward [8]. For example, is the child attending a school in which their ethnic minority is perceived positively as a group? Are they, themselves, a majority group in their own community? Both of these circumstances may move an individual more toward greater exploration and commitment to their own ethnicity. But how fluid is identity after all, especially for an adolescent? For adolescents, "identity" and allegiances may change according to the specific context that they are in (e.g., "code switching" [2] or "hybrid identities" [3]); it may be important for the clinician to determine how fluid or how static their sense of identity may be.

It is likely that many older adolescents are moving toward the "achieved" identity status, which includes integrating all the many aspects of identity and forming a strong hybrid identity. These are the adolescents that are likely to manifest a great deal of resiliency. What determines the ability to integrate and remain resilient in the face of acculturative stress as well as the role hybrid identities may have in youth identity development are still questions that deserve much attention.

Importance of Acculturation Assessment

Acculturation Gap: The Role of Children

When parents and children cannot see "eye-to-eye", difficulties and conflict can arise. Ying and Han [10] found that in a sample of Southeast Asian American teens, adolescents' perceived generational/cultural gap (as mediated by conflict) was related to rates of depression. More specifically, greater conflict was related to higher rates of depression. Another study found that in Asian American families, a perceived autocratic parenting style by adolescents (high level of control and little warmth) was related to higher rates of depression in girls [11]. The amount of conflict was measured and used to validate parenting style, which means that there was a fair amount of conflict likely present in the perceived autocratic parenting families. Rhee et al. [12] found that Asian American teens have reported higher levels of self-esteem if there is less perceived conflict between them and their parents. And finally, Hahm et al. [13] found that even with more highly acculturated adolescents (or more Western identified adolescents), parental attachment was a significant mediator in alcohol use, meaning that the more attached they were to their parents, the less alcohol they used. In summary, it is important to perform an ongoing assessment of the acculturation gap, intergenerational conflict, and even attachment from both the perspective of the parent as well as the perspective of the child in helping determine what influence it may play in the child's mental health.

---

[2] Linguistics and education refer to "code switching" as the use of two or more languages within a single conversation or the use of different manners of speaking and interacting that are dependent on the context in which the individual is operating (e.g., conversations with close friends vs. in the classroom).

[3] In emerging literature on culturally responsive education, "hybrid identity" refers to the multifaceted understanding of identity in a sociocultural context [9]. It addresses how identity is understood as well as expressed or enacted by individuals. For example, for immigrant youth in some urban and rural areas, how the youth identifies with components of both the majority group as well as other minority groups with which they interact are important influences on how strongly they identify with their own ethnic group and the extent to which their identities may blend aspects of other ethnic identities into their own.

Acculturation Gap: The Role of Parents

The parent/child culture gap can lead to many difficulties for both parents and children in the acculturation process. For parents, particular aspects of the "gap" may include parenting practices and beliefs that are not consistent with their child's beliefs (e.g., infrequent praise and affection), lack of knowledge of development in both the home and host countries, and differences in expectations about their children. Many parents will subscribe to the parenting expectations with which they are familiar. For example, many Korean parents believe that corporal punishment is necessary when disciplining children [14]. Another example is that in a sample of Japanese parents, it was found that most believed effort is much more important to the success of their children than ability, especially given negative outcomes [15]. Parenting beliefs and behaviors may change as parents acculturate; they may begin to look more like the host culture's beliefs. But parents may continue to struggle with which parenting practices to choose. This is compounded by their shaken confidence in parenting due to asymmetrical acculturation. It has been found that Chinese mothers who perceived a large acculturation gap between themselves and their children had more parenting difficulties as measured by difficulties in communication and in overall satisfaction in their relationship [16]. In addition, in another study, it was found that the more acculturated mothers were, the more attenuated or fewer difficulties were reported in the psychological adjustment of their children [17].

To add to the complication, there may be differences between the acculturative changes between members of parenting dyads (intragenerational), which may also lead to additional conflict and difficulties for the families. Fathers may be out in the work force, learning English and American behaviors faster than wives, but wives may have more exposure to their acculturating children, schools, and have a greater empathy for their children's acculturative process. It is well known from forensic studies and divorce cases that parental conflict is one of the most important determinants of a child's well being, for example, high parental conflict, greater distress in the child [18]. It can therefore be concluded that conflict in any parenting unit would lead to difficulties in children.

An additional consideration in parental influence on their child's mental health is the child's perception of how accepting their parents are of them. A Korean study found that adolescent's perceptions of how much their parents accepted them were correlated to their psychological adjustment [19]. Perceptions by children as well as by parents are unquestionably critical in determining the emotional well-being of both as these previous studies demonstrate.

Parental Psychopathology and Impact on Children

It has long been known that when parents struggle, their children also tend to struggle. It is therefore critical for every clinician to consider both the emotional health of the parent and how it impacts their ability to parent, their self-esteem as a capable parent, and, finally, how mental illness is perceived by their home country as well as their willingness to seek out help. Parental self-esteem is especially important to consider given that there is the common phenomenology of "role reversal" between immigrant parents and children. It can be very demoralizing to have to depend on a child for very fundamental things (e.g., talking to teachers about school performance, paying bills, or visiting the doctor). As it has been noted previously, many Asian cultures are hierarchical in nature and Confucianism is still commonly practiced in many Asian families. Thus, it can be especially challenging for parents to depend on their children and still feel self-assured and competent. Because of this difficulty, it is not uncommon for Asian American parents to struggle with such things as depression, anxiety, and low self-esteem.

The impact of depression on mothers and fathers can influence such things as parenting, disciplining practices, and the emotional well-being of their children. Despite the popular belief that Asians and Asian Americans have low rates of depression, Huang et al. [20] found that the rates of depression among foreign-born mothers were relatively low compared with US-born mothers, except in the case of Asian mothers. Foreign-born mothers, *including* Asian mothers, were also more likely to believe that they did not have to seek help for their depression. McLearn et al. [21] found that mothers of infants were not as safety conscious or as interactive when they were depressed themselves.[4] They were also found to have increased odds of using harsher forms of discipline (e.g., corporal punishment). Kim and Ge [22] found that adolescent depressive symptoms were related to their perceptions of harsh discipline and disrupted parenting practices in Chinese American families.

If one considers the stresses of the Asian American immigrant family, then there are several additional acculturative variables to assess when working with Asian American children. For example, Fenton et al. [23] describe how there were four Asian infants that had failure to thrive because of maternal isolation, inability to communicate to seek help, and denial on the father's part that there was a problem to acknowledge. In a study in Hong Kong, Shek [24] found that in Chinese families, paternal qualities were more related to adolescent psychological well-being than maternal qualities. This last-mentioned study highlights not only the universality of parental influence on child and adolescent well-being but also the importance of considering what role each parent plays in their child's life, the dynamic between parents, what life was like for their families in their home countries, how their countries perceived mental illness and how their communities/families dealt with it, what was culturally sanctioned and what was condemned, and how this has all changed or remained constant for them and their families since beginning their lives in a different country. Their mental health/mental illness beliefs will be just as important to assess as other behaviors, beliefs, and practices, for these will also change as they acculturate.

---

[4] It should be noted that this study used a non-Asian sample.

Psychopathology in Asian Children and Adolescents

Despite studies that suggest that Asian American children and adolescents have lower rates of psychiatric illness [25–27], there has been increasing evidence to suggest that the opposite is true and that both internalizing and externalizing diagnoses are warranted in Asian American children and teens. Recently, there are certain behaviors/diagnoses that have received more attention by researchers and clinicians in Asian children and adolescents, which include the following: depression, somatic presentations of distress, anxiety, suicide, substance abuse, and disruptive behavior/delinquency. Some of this recent research literature will be presented in the following sections.

Somatized Distress

It is known that Asian and Asian American patients may tend to focus more on physical symptoms of discomfort or pain rather than on emotional distress upon their initial clinical visits. However, for many Asian patients, they are often fully aware of socioemotional stress in their lives. When asked specifically about these psychological symptoms, it has been shown that they have had little difficulty reporting these feelings [28]. Although several of these studies do not distinguish between degrees of acculturation and generational level, it is important to consider the influence of the "culturally bound acceptance" of psychological dysfunction by the patient and its influence on reporting of these symptoms. Thus, brief mention is made here with regard to somatic complaints in Asian children and adolescents. Choi et al. [29] found that in Korean American youth, somatic complaints were highly correlated with depression. Children, depending on age, might present somatically regardless of the level of acculturation. As noted previously, it would be important to then consider the level of acculturation of parents or caregivers as they will often times determine when to seek help for their children.

Depression

The rates for anxiety and depression across ethnicities seem to be similar, although there may be more controversy surrounding the rates for depression in Asian American adolescents [30, 31]. One possible reason is that culture and ethnicity influence diagnostic bias in diverse ethnicities of adolescents [4]. Thus, based on the limitations of available diagnostic tools as well as influences on diagnostic bias, it is assumed by many clinicians that Asian American children and teens have low rates of depression because they are the "model minority." However, due to the expected obedience to adults and a lack of wanting to bring disgrace to their families, the likelihood of a somatized presentation of depression, and/or the lack of understanding by the adults in their lives, Asian youth may be more reluctant to share feelings of depression. Furthermore, children and adolescents may also feel defective which may additionally fuel feelings of inadequacy or guilt. For example, it has been found that Koreans tend to believe that depression is simply a lack of motivation or a lack of trying on the child's part [33]. With regard to academic achievement, Kim reported that both perfectionist traits and perceived criticism from parents were found to be related to depression. In addition, a study of second-generation Chinese American adolescents found levels of reported stress (e.g., from academic life), higher levels of depression [34].

It has also been shown that generational status (which generation someone is when they migrate) can influence the presentation of dysfunction. For example, Willgerodt and Thompson [35] found that in a sample of Filipino, Chinese, and European-descended adolescents, generational status (e.g., first, second, or multiple generation) was predictive of somatic symptoms and substance use. This was in addition to ethnicity being predictive of depression and delinquency scores. More specifically, Filipino adolescents had the highest rates of depression and delinquency, and higher-generation Asian American adolescents had more somatic complaints and substance abuse than second- or first-generation adolescents. The finding that somatic complaints were found to be higher in potentially more acculturated Asian adolescents is perplexing, although authors of this particular study wonder if it is due to the more specific delineation among ethnicities (which has not necessarily been the case in previous studies).

All of these studies highlight the importance of trying to determine the influence of particular factors – ethnicity, generation, relationship with family, expectations regarding academic performance, diagnostic criteria, the use of diagnostic screens and scales, micro- and macrocultural context, and other more specific issues – on the psychosocial well-being of Asian American children and adolescents.

Anxiety

There are several types of anxiety that are relevant when discussing Asian American children and adolescents. In a study by Austin and Chorpita [31], a group of Native Hawaiian, Filipino, Chinese, Japanese, and European American children and adolescents were sampled; they found that there were interethnic differences in the rates of anxiety and that there were differences in rates depending on which kind of anxiety was evaluated. In their study, Native Hawaiian children and teens (grades 3rd–12th) scored highest for separation anxiety and Chinese children and teens scored highest for social phobia. Although they did not collect data regarding generational status or acculturative level, these variables may help explain which kinds of anxiety are likely to be relevant. For example, it has been found that Chinese children and adolescents in China have high rates of social anxiety evaluated from the ages of 11–13 years of age due to the structure of the education system in China and the pressure at that developmental age to achieve academically [36]. Therefore, it may be important to consider how recently the child has immigrated from their home country to help shed light on the etiology of dysfunction.

There has also been limited work exploring the link between self-identity/identity formation and anxiety. For example, do mixed race/ethnicity individuals have higher rates of anxiety than non-mixed race/ethnicity individuals? In a study by Williams et al. [37], which included Japanese and mixed-race Japanese American adolescents, no significant relationships were found between gender or generation and anxiety levels. They did find, however, that the Japanese American teens had lower rates of anxiety compared to the mixed-race Japanese American teens. The authors speculate that part of this reason is due to difficulties in identity formation in the mixed ethnicity children and possibly the lower amount of fidelity to one specific ethnic group.

Suicide

Asian American youths are also at risk for suicide despite the common belief that suicide and suicidal ideation in this population are low. It is likely that there is an underestimation of the rate of suicidal ideation as it may never come to the attention of others. The difficulties in help-seeking behaviors may be due to the fear of shaming their families and themselves, reluctance in sharing distress with parents, admitting to "weakness" in needing counseling, and denying or not recognizing the difficulties that they might be struggling with.

Specific risk factors for suicidal ideation in Asian American youth are acculturation stresses, particularly, identity confusion or failure to successfully navigate a bicultural identity, academic stressors, discrimination, and parental conflict [38, 39]. Alienation due to culture or cultural conflict has also been cited to be risk factors [40, 41]. It has been found that the rates of suicide among foreign-born Asian youth are higher than for American-born Asian Youth [39, 42]. It is important to mention at this juncture that the rates of suicide in China are three times the global average with girls between 15–24 years being particularly vulnerable [43]. This highlights the importance of assessing multiple risk factors (e.g. gender, stresses in one's host culture and stresses in one's new culture) and determining what role each may play in one's distress.

To further demonstrate the possible link between academic stress and suicidal ideation, in 2005, Cornell University's Asian and Asian American Campus Climate Taskforce (3ATF) found that although Asian and Asian Americans comprised 17% of the student population (notably, also the largest community of color on campus), 50% of completed suicides at the school had been committed by this student population [44, 45]. In addition, the findings also noted that Asian and Asian American students were less likely to utilize campus counseling services. However, they tended to report having issues with sleep, a sense of hopelessness and stress in addition to abuse in relationships more often. Although this example focuses on college-age Asian American students, it is important to remember that the issues that led to these difficulties likely began earlier.

Substance Abuse

In the past, it has been surmised or stated by many researchers and clinicians alike that Asian American adolescents do not abuse drugs as much as other ethnic/race adolescents [46, 47]. Many of these studies usually sample several different non-Asian ethnic groups, including European American, African American, and Latino American. In several of these studies, no distinctions are made among the different Asian ethnicities and there is no assessment of acculturative stage, in addition to many other factors such as parental relationship, identity, etc. When these factors are accounted for, different conclusions are reached.

In the National Youth Tobacco Survey (NYTS) 2000 data on tobacco use in youth, it was found that one-third of the Asian American youth surveyed were smokers [48]. Further examination of the NYTS 2000 data also showed that the tobacco use rates increased as Asian American/Pacific Islander youth aged [49]. It has also been shown that there are differential rates of smoking in different ethnicities within the "Asian American" categorization. For example, in a sample surveyed in Hawaii, it was found that smoking rates among Native Hawaiian/Pacific Islander and Filipino students were highest, and rates of smoking of Japanese and Chinese students were lowest [50]. With regard to drinking, research has shown that Koreans had rates of binge drinking that were four times greater than their Chinese counterparts and were also greater than the rates reported for other Asian groups [33].[5] These examples highlight the need for differential consideration for the differences in ethnicity in our clinical work.

Another factor that is important to consider is the level of acculturation and its impact on familial relationships. Hahm et al. [13] found that the greater the level of acculturation, the greater the alcohol use in Asian American adolescents. However, parental attachment was a mediating factor. For example, if the adolescents were highly attached to their parents, then they had no greater risk than those adolescents who were less acculturated. Once again, this emphasizes the crucial need to determine the nature of the relationship between the adolescent and parent and what impact it has on the presenting dysfunction.

---

[5] It should be noted that this study focused on a college-age sample.

It would be important to mention here as well that many of the studies on Asian American children and adolescents do not fully assess for full acculturative level and relationship to identity. As noted earlier, one can be highly identified to Western culture and not to Asian culture. Do these adolescents fair more poorly and have more psychopathology than the adolescents that are highly identified with both Asian and Western culture? James et al. [51] looked at the link between adolescent ethnic identity and drug use. They determined that high ethnic identity was related to higher levels of drug use. Level of identification with the host culture was not assessed. Once again, there is great importance in thinking critically about how the adolescent identifies themselves and its link to self-esteem, what their relationships look like with their parents as well as their friends, which Asian group they identify with most, the levels of acculturation of both children and parents, how the information is obtained and whether or not there is minimization present in addition to what other stressors might be relevant, and what psychopathology might be co-morbid.

Externalized Behaviors: Delinquency and Gang-Related Activity

Differential effects of ethnicity and acculturative level have also been found to influence youth violence and delinquent behaviors. A study that looked at the rates of youth violence in Hawaii found that Filipino, Hawaiian, and Samoan youth all had higher rates of delinquent behaviors than the Japanese group sampled [52]. At this juncture, it is important to note that the history of a group and the particular history of the individual presenting, especially in their particular environment, may be critical to consider when performing an assessment.[6] In this study, although the Japanese group was a relatively new group to the island, they have still been there for generations, which likely implies that acculturative stressors may not be as relevant for this group as a whole as it would be for the more recently immigrated Southeast Asians, for example. It is well known that Native Hawaiian and Pacific Islanders tend to fare poorly with regard to health outcomes relative to the other ethnicities on the island. In this situation, ethnicity and the history of the group likely played a more important role in the delinquency outcomes than the "newness" of the group. Is it more than

---

[6] It would be prudent to mention that the Asian population in Hawaii is 41.5% according to the 2005 census as compared with the 4.3% found in the United States overall. The percentage of Native Hawaiian and other Pacific Islander (Guam, Samoa, or other Pacific Islands) is 9.0% as compared with the 0.2% found in the United States [53]. There was a wave of migration by Japanese and Chinese immigrants to Hawaii in the nineteenth century for work, for example, as "cheap labor" for the large plantations. These populations have been on the Island for several decades; thus, there are multiple-generation Asians present now on Hawaii in addition to new generations. The Native Hawaiian/Pacific Islander population has been found to have worse health outcomes than the rest of the population of the United States, likely due to disparities and barriers in access to health care [54].

coincidence that the adolescents in these groups have chosen more externalized ways of expressing distress than internalized? This is yet another question to consider when looking forward to how our research can better guide our clinical work.

With regard to delinquency, Erikson (1, p. 132) stated that:

> Youth after youth, bewildered by the incapacity to assume a role forced on him by the inexorable standardization of American adolescence, runs away in one form or another, dropping out of school, leaving jobs, staying out all night, or withdrawing into bizarre and inaccessible moods. Once "delinquent," his greatest need and often his only salvation is the refusal on the part of older friends, advisers, and judiciary personnel to type him further... It is here... that the concept of identity confusion is of practical clinical value...

Some clinicians may work under the assumption that delinquency in Asian American youth is linked to uninvolved parenting. On the contrary, Goldberg [55] found that in a sample of Cambodian students who all had serious problems with truancy, these students' reports indicated this was not the case. Instead, it was found that when a bilingual Cambodian worker at the school conducted outreach phone calls, many of the parents were very eager to learn more about the school's expectations and practices and about their child's academic performance. Cambodian youth in this study reported that the most important reasons for their truant behavior included involvement with drugs, pressure from peers, and involvement with gangs. Boredom and the need for socializing with friends were given as next in importance. With regard to street- or gang-involved youth, it is important to note, that it is not necessarily the expectation or peer pressure from other gang members to skip school, but more the "hanging out" lifestyle (e.g., staying out until 2 AM) that is most compelling.

It has been suggested by some that more culturally sensitive interventions need to be implemented, for example, such as with the issue of truancy. Goldberg [55] suggested interventions for use with truant Cambodian youth to include providing opportunities for "friendship groups," making academic work more personally relevant and interesting to the students, and helping students explore how negative activities outside of school affect the individual's functioning in school. In addition, providing culturally and linguistically sensitive opportunities for parents to engage in and learn more about the school process and their child's progress was considered essential. Clinicians may be able to provide valuable consultation to the schools to address the incredibly difficult situations such as truancy and other delinquent behaviors.

Special Mention of Interethnic Dating and Gender/Sexuality Issues

It is significant to note that increased proximity and engagement with "American" communities (e.g., neighborhoods and schools) play a part in increasing the likelihood of opportunities for relationships between different ethnic and racial groups [56, 57]. As noted previously, children are making decisions regarding their romantic partners without the input of their parents which is not traditional practice in many Asian countries.

Outdating or outmarrying[7] in many ways contradicts long-held Asian traditions as it downplays the importance of family in continuation of the family blood line and preservation of traditional family and cultural values held dear in many households [58]. As a result, issues of interethnic or interracial dating and marriage can heighten both intergenerational and cultural conflict between parents and children. Consideration of the parents' attitudes and personal experiences with interracial coupling and other ethnicities (e.g., US military occupations or personal experiences with individuals) must be taken into account when understanding intercultural and intergenerational conflict with children regarding this matter. It is not uncommon to have arguments spanning years over the choice of spouse, which can definitely take a toll on the well-being of both individuals and their families.

In addition, sexual minority youth – lesbian, gay, bisexual, transgender, and intersexual (LGBTI) – face a multitude of problems that include "feelings of isolation, negative family reaction, verbal and physical abuse, sexual abuse, sexually transmitted diseases, poor school performance, mental health problems, substance abuse, running away, and conflict with the law" (59, pp. 159–160). Chung and Katayama [59] argued that in modern-day society, although general attitudes toward homosexuality are similar in both Asian and Western cultures, "the intensity of heterosexism and homophobia is much stronger in Asian cultures than in American" (59, p. 163) because of the intersection of homophobia and traditional Asian values, which often emphasize the importance of continuing the family name and blood line.

The double-minority status – ethnic minority and sexual minority – for Asian and Asian Pacific American LGBTI youth highlights the possible complexity of simultaneous cultural and sexual identity development. The ultimate goal is for Asian Pacific American LGBTI's to achieve integration of both identities. Unfortunately, for many, having a high Asian identity often means facing great obstacles in building a strong sexual identity because of cultural issues of homophobia and heterosexism. Any young man or woman, however, with a strong sexual identity will also most likely face barriers in developing an integrated ethnic identity because of issues of racism and intracultural shame [59]. For Asian Americans, "choosing one's sexual gender identity often means losing the safety net against racism and cultural insensitivity from their ethnic community" (60, p. 60). Thus, clinicians are in a unique position to gain deeper understanding and referral of culturally sensitive types of support available for Asian LGBTI (e.g., the Gay Asian

---

[7] Outdating or outmarrying refers to the marriage to or dating of persons outside of one's own ethnic or racial group.

Pacific Support Network) in addressing issues of both acculturation and sexual identity, as they relate to the mental health of the individual Asian Pacific American LGBTI youth.

Risk Factors and Resiliency

Emerging research from the youth development field notes that there are a number of protective factors that can be present or can be fortified in a young person's life that helps to better support them as they navigate difficult periods [32, 61]. But what determines who of our immigrant youth will struggle with mental health issues? With regard to resiliency, there is reason to believe that this is affected by a number of factors such as acculturative status, ethnicity, gender, identity, religious affiliation, education level, socioeconomic status (SES) of the parents, relationship to parents, and perceived family support. And as we have seen, some of these factors can be either a risk factor or a strength given the particular situation or their interactions with other factors present. Although research is limited in assessing resiliency factors specifically in Asian American children and their families, some studies as mentioned earlier have been successful in demonstrating what factors may be protective.

With regard to risk and protective factors, it is important to reiterate that family conflict (intergenerational conflict between children and parents) is one of the main risk factors for psychopathology and dysfunction. Therefore, good relationships between children and their parents are likely protective. A study looking at Filipino adolescents in Hawaii found that family support was protective against academic and emotional difficulties [62]. However, also in this study, it was found that lower SES of the parents was correlated with poorer mental health outcomes in the children. In another study performed in a minority, but non-Asian sample, it was found that diffuse ethnic identity and perceived discrimination were risk factors. Family values and bicultural competence were protective factors [63]. Interestingly, they also found that first-generation girls and second-generation boys were at particular risk for emotional difficulties, which indicates that gender and generation may interact to pose specific increased risk.

A brief mention is made here with regard to religion and its relationship to distress in Asian families. Many Asian immigrants subscribe and practice religion of some sort, from Buddhism to Catholicism. It has been found that specific aspects of religion or religious practice can be either risk or protective factors in Asian adults [64]. For example, loci of control factors were differentially related to distress in European Americans vs. Korean Americans. It was found that Korean Americans found more relief (and a lower rate of depression) in believing that God controlled events vs. European Americans who found less relief. However, it was related to higher rates of anxiety in Korean Americans [65]. This was a study performed using an adult sample, which likely means that these findings might be more relevant for the parents of the children with whom we work. Until we have more studies to assess coping in children and adolescents, we may judiciously use these adult studies as possible hypotheses as they may be helpful in informing our work with children and their families.

How do Children and Adolescents Come to Our Attention and What to Consider in Evaluation and Treatment

It is well known that often Asian American children and adolescents will not present to the therapist's office or the psychiatrist's office initially and are instead referred by schools, pediatricians, child welfare agencies, and other referral sources. Families may come to the attention of mental health practitioners reluctantly, with great shame, denial of any difficulties, and anger toward the entities that provided referral. It is important to consider this when approaching an Asian family in the clinical setting. Once again, it is likely that the level of acculturation will be critical to consider in the assessment. For example, if the parents/caregivers as well as the child or adolescent subscribes to more Westernized practices, it is possible to find no more reluctance for treatment than the "typical" American patient. But if the family is not very Westernized, or if the parents are not very Westernized but the children are more so, then the practitioner should be prepared to utilize different methods of assessment and engagement. The clinician should expect different manifestations of the presenting chief complaints and how psychological distress is communicated. All of this may require different or multifaceted treatment plans for optimal engagement and treatment of the Asian American patient and their family. Some considerations are as follows:

Clinical Considerations When Working with Children and Adolescents: General Thoughts

1. Determine who is doing the referral and why – not all families will identify that there is a problem (because of lack of information, shame, lack of communication, etc.)
2. It is likely they will not be coming to *your* office; you may have to work within the school context, for example, as a consultant, or in a pediatrician's office if families are reluctant to come to seek the help of a mental health practitioner. Thus, collaborative care is essential and includes determining who plays what role in the assessment and treatment over time.

3. If language is a barrier, find someone to provide professional language/cultural translation. One can also consider the use of collateral sources (e.g., interpretation telephone lines or community-based organizations[8]). If these are not readily available, then ask parents if they might know someone who could help (e.g., reverend/minister at church, trusted community leader, relative, or friend). It is important to be aware that this will not be an option for some who are members of small ethnic communities due to shame and fear of judgment. As a last resort, one may consider using children, although it is not recommended, as this can come with further shame and role reversal of parents. In addition, children knowing about parent's beliefs and wishes for the child may not be ideal. Also, be aware that some parents may reject or refuse to use interpreters because of embarrassment or fear. Although it is important to be respectful of their wishes, it is also important to communicate when you believe that a case would ideally warrant interpreter services. Try to normalize the use of interpreters and possibly explore with the parents further what the use of interpreters means to them.
4. It is always critical to obtain the parent's perspective and experience – if they do not perceive a problem, determine whether there truly is a problem with the child or adolescent (e.g., referral source lacking understanding of culture). If it is difficulty in cultural expectations by the referral source, then provide culturally specific psychoeducation. If there is a possible identified problem, but the parents are primary contributors (e.g., corporal punishment or parent-initiated conflict), then consider a sensitive referral that will meet their needs.
5. Identify the level of acculturation for both parents and children, the amount of conflict, the amount of distress each party perceives (e.g., parents and child), and how much their perspectives differ; do not forget that each parent could also have a different acculturative perspective. One may consider using screens such as the ones mentioned in this book. Determine how acculturative level and conflict influence the presenting (or nonpresenting) problems. For example, is the child being bullied/discriminated against at school for not speaking English fluently (acculturative stress)? Have the parents determined the child is "bad" for not listening to them at home (acculturative conflict)?
6. Determine how the assessment should proceed and be flexible; children may not divulge abuse at home, and parents may not allow the child to be assessed alone. Try to elicit worry from parents (e.g., if acting out at school or failing academic performance) and normalize the manner in which the interview occurs. Building an alliance may be the primary focus for the first several visits.

---

[8] Community or faith-based organizations may have counselors or other qualified professional staff on hand who can assist in translation, although one must be sensitive to the parent/guardian's feelings toward seeking help from organizations or persons who may be part of their own ethnic communities.

7. Evaluate the quality of previous experiences with mental health vs. current mental health experiences and the family's perceptions of these experiences.
8. If there is a family conflict problem, then one may consider providing recommendations for interventions such as the ones mentioned earlier in this volume (e.g. Strengthening Intergenerational/Intercultural Ties in Immigrant Families), family therapy, or some form of therapy that respects the nature of the family relationships. One may additionally consider the use of home-based teams or family–community liaison for parents to reestablish authority and navigate their communities successfully without being dependent on their children. It is also important to determine what role each parent plays in the child's life and to use this information to guide assessment and treatment planning.
9. Always consider the child's perspective as unique and valuable. Provide culturally appropriate toys and games when applicable (e.g., if the child is not very American culture-identified).
10. Determine the acculturative level of parents and consider matching parents with a specific therapeutic style (e.g., approaching parents with more authoritarian recommendations if recently immigrated). Remember that you are likely to perform work with parents in addition to work with the child.
11. Assess for comparisons made between the "model" child, for example, a sibling who is excelling academically and your patient and consider how they are impacting the well-being of your child. Observation of and processing this dynamic may be part of the work with your patient as well as their family.
12. Assess the developmental stage (in both home country and Western schema) and try to determine where the child falls in the spectrum. Also, consider the interaction between the two cultures (e.g., how are they similar or dissimilar), the history of the family as well as the group in their new country, and how these may influence development. Determine if their behaviors or difficulties may be some interaction between acculturation and development (e.g., when a child is not speaking at expected age in a bilingual home).
13. Do not ignore your own comfort with the case, the work with the family, and your own biases/limitations/history. These can all influence the working relationship, the process, and the outcomes of any given case. Also, it is important to be aware of your own tendencies for overidentification (either with child or parents), under or overattribution of dysfunction to culture, or any assumptions made especially if you are from a similar cultural background.

Work with Adolescents

1. Assess for such things as bullying/discrimination or racism (e.g., being victimized), sexuality issues, interracial relationships, suicidal ideation, or other things that they may be more reluctant to share with either you or their parents.

2. It will be important to figure out how acculturated the adolescent is, where family is, and if there is a large gap in clinical expectations. For example, if the adolescent is much more Westernized than their parents, then they might want to meet with the clinician alone to have more confidentiality. If parents are much more traditional, this might pose great difficulties. Clinicians may find themselves feeling "caught" and may lose rapport with either or both. One may try to recognize the dilemma with both the parents and the adolescents, normalize the dilemma, and try to figure out (preferably with the entire family's involvement) how best to proceed. Also, it may be important to acknowledge and admit to your own limitations.
3. Determine whether there is an active process of identity formation and, if already consolidated, what their identity comprises such as ethnic/group affiliation, sexual orientation, and gender identity, etc. It will also be important to determine how identity issues may be related to the presenting difficulties. In the case of an adolescent with a more marginalized or diffuse identity, it may be necessary to incorporate the work of identity integration.
4. The adolescent may want treatment and the parents may not and vice versa. Attempt to work with both, validating the parents' role in the life of the adolescent and in determining whether treatment can proceed.
5. If there are concerns about interracial relationships/LGBTI issues, the treatment should include both education and empathic recognition of the difficulties for both parents and children. It is important to gain a deeper understanding about how these issues are perceived within one's home culture and how these expectations and assumptions influence intergenerational conflict. Providing appropriate referral to supportive organizations may be recommended for either the parents or the child.
6. For delinquency issues, immigrant families typically lack knowledge about and access to American educational and legal systems. Consider connecting families with appropriate culturally/linguistically sensitive school liaisons, with organizations who specialize in assiting families in legal or educational advocacy, and provide consultation when appropriate to these organizations about Asian-specific acculturative issues.

Conclusion

There is a desperate need for more evidence-based research to inform clinical decision-making when working with Asian American children and adolescents. Meanwhile, a combination of existing research findings as well as thoughtful clinical practice can provide guidelines that help clinicians feel less daunted by the task of working with a language or culture that is unfamiliar. On account of the recent waves of immigration by Asian families and the resultant time spent here in the United States, we as clinicians are now being faced with the ever-growing issue of addressing the acculturation stressors and conflicts in the lives of our patients. Hopefully, we can continue to effectively collaborate and learn from the families and the communities with which we work and allow this work to help us be more sensitive to all children, adolescents, and families.

References

1. Erikson E. Identity: youth and crisis. New York: Norton; 1968.
2. Chu MM, Lee WC, Leung JLS, Wong V. Modified symbolic play test for oriental children. Pediatr Int 2006;48:519–524.
3. Park MS. The factors of child physical abuse in Korean families. Child Abuse Negl 2001;25:945–958.
4. Choi H. Understanding adolescent depression in ethnocultural context. Adv Nurs Sci 2002;25(2):71–85.
5. Louie VS. Compelled to excel: immigration, education, and opportunity among Chinese Americans. Stanford, CA: Stanford University Press; 2004
6. Marcia J. Identity in adolescence. In: Adelson J, editor. Handbook of adolescent psychology. New York: Wiley; 1980, pp. 159–187.
7. Phinney JS. Stages of ethnic identity in minority group adolescents. J Early Adolesc 1989;19:34–49.
8. Umaña-Taylor AJ. Ethnic identity and self-esteem: examining the role of social context. J Adolesc 2004;27:139–46.
9. Irizarry J. Ethnic and urban intersections in the classroom: Latino students, hybrid identities, and culturally responsive pedagogy. Multicult Perspect 2007;9(3):21–28.
10. Ying YW, Han M. The longitudinal effect of intergenerational gap in acculturation on conflict and mental health in Southeast Asian American adolescents. Am J Orthopsychiatry 2007;77(1):61–66.
11. Radziszewska B, Richardson BL, Dent CW, Flay BR. Parenting style and adolescent depressive symptoms, smoking, and academic achievement: ethnic, gender, and SES differences. J Behav Med 1996;19(3):289–305.
12. Rhee S, Chang J, Rhee J. Acculturation, communication patterns, and self-esteem among Asian and Caucasian American adolescents. Adolescence 2003;38(152):749–768.
13. Hahm HC, Lahiff M, Guterman NB. Acculturation and parental attachment in Asian-American adolescents' alcohol use. J Adolesc Health 2003;33:119–129.
14. Chun BH. Child abuse in Korea. Child Welfare 1989;68:154–158.
15. Bornstein MH, Cote LR. Mother's parenting cognitions in cultures of origin, acculturating cultures, and cultures of destination. Child Dev 2004;75(1):221–235.
16. Buki LP, Ma TC, Strom RD, Strom SK. Chinese immigrant mothers of adolescents self-perceptions of acculturation effects on parenting. Cultur Divers Ethnic Minor Psychol 2003;9(2):127–140.
17. Kim E, Cain K, McCubbin M. Maternal and paternal parenting, acculturation, and young adolescents' psychological adjustment. J Child Adolesc Psychiatr Nurs 2006;19(3). 112–129.
18. Kelly JB. Marital conflict, divorce, and children's adjustment. Child Adolesc Psychiatr Clin N Am 1998;7(2):259–271.
19. Kim E, Han G, McCubbin MA. Korean American maternal acceptance-rejection, acculturation, and children's social competence. Fam Community Health 2007;30(2 Suppl): 33–45.
20. Huang ZJ, Wong FY, Ronzio CR, Yu SM. Depressive symptomatology and mental health help-seeking patterns of US and foreign-born mothers. Matern Child Health J 2007 May;11(3):257–267.

21. McLearn KT, Minkovitz CS, Strobino DM, Marks E, Hou W. The timing of maternal depressive symptoms and mothers' parenting practices with young children; implications for pediatric practice. Pediatrics 2006;118(1):174–182.
22. Kim SY, Ge X. Parenting practices and adolescent depressive symptoms in Chinese American families. J Fam Psychol 2000 Sept;14(3):420–35.
23. Fenton TR, Bhat R, Davies A, West R. Maternal insecurity and failure to thrive in Asian children. Arch Dis Child 1989;64(3):369–372.
24. Shek DT. Paternal and maternal influences on the psychological well-being of Chinese adolescents. Genet Soc Gen Psychol Monogr 1999;125(3):269–296.
25. Roberts RE, Roberts CR, Chen YR. Ethnocultural differences in adolescent depression. Am J Community Psychol 1997;25(1):95–110.
26. Chen IG, Roberts RE, Aday LA. Ethnicity and adolescent depression: the case of Chinese Americans. J Nerv Ment Dis 1998 Oct;186(10):623–630.
27. Guaio IZ, Thompson EA. Ethnicity and problem behaviors among adolescent females in the United States. Health Care Women Int 2004 Apr;25(4):296–310.
28. Lin KM, Cheung F. Mental health issues for Asian Americans. Psychiatr Serv 1999;50(6): 774–780.
29. Choi H, Stafford L, Meininger JC, Roberts, RE, Smith DP. Psychometric properties of the DSM scale for depression (DSD) with Korean-American youths. Issues Ment Health Nurs 2002;23(8):735–756.
30. Gee CB. Assessment of anxiety and depression in Asian American youth. J Clin Child Adolesc Psychol 2004 Jun;33(2):269–271.
31. Austin AA, Chorpita BF. Temperament, anxiety, and depression: comparisons across five ethnic groups of children. J Clin Child Adolesc Psychol 2004;33(2):216–226.
32. Land H, Levy A. A school-based prevention model for depressed Asian adolescents. Soc Work Educ 1992;14(3):165–176.
33. Kim JM. Culture-specific psychoeducational induction talk as an intervention to increase service utilization amongst minority populations: the case of Korean Americans. American Counseling Association. In: Walz GR, Yep RK, editors. VISTAS: compelling perspectives on counseling 2005. Portland, OR: Book News, Inc.; 2005, pp. 129–132.
34. Jose PE, Huntsinger CS. Moderation and mediation effects of coping by Chinese American and European American adolescents. J Genet Psychol 2005;166(1):16–43.
35. Willgerodt MA, Thompson EA. Ethnic and generational influences on emotional distress and risk behaviors among Chinese and Filipino American adolescents. Res Nurs Health 2006 Aug;29(4):311–324.
36. Dong Q, Yang B, Ollendick TH. Fears in Chinese children and adolescents and their relations to anxiety and depression. J Child Psychol Psychiatr 1994;35(2):351–363.
37. Williams JK, Goebert D, Hishinuma E, Miyamoto R, Anzai N, Izutsu S, et al.. A conceptual model of cultural predictors of anxiety among Japanese American and part-Japanese American adolescents. Cultur Divers Ethnic Minor Psychol 2002;8(4): 320–333.
38. Groves SA, Stanley BH, Sher L. Ethnicity and the relationship between adolescent alcohol use and suicidal behavior. Int J Adolesc Med Health 2007;19(1):19–25.
39. Lau AS, Jernewall NM, Zane N, Myers HF. Correlates of suicidal behaviors among Asian American outpatient youth. Cultur Divers Ethnic Minor Psychol 2002;8(3): 199–213.
40. Bhugra D. Suicidal behavior in South Asians in the UK. Crisis 2002;23(3):108–113.
41. Handy S, Chithiramohan RN, Ballard CG, Silveira WR. Ethnic differences in adolescent self-poisoning; a comparison of Asian and Caucasian groups. J Adolesc 1991;14(2): 157–162.
42. Liu WT, Yu ES, Chang C, Fernandez M. The mental health of Asian American teenagers: a research challenge. In: Stiffman AR, Davis LE, editors. Ethnic issues in adolescent mental health. Newbury Park, CA: Sage; 1990, p. 92–112.

43. Hesketh T, Ding QJ, Jenkins R. Suicide ideation in Chinese adolescents. Soc Psychiatry Psychiatr Epidemiol 2002;37(5):230–35.
44. Harder L. Asian Americans commit half of suicides at Cornell. The Cornell Daily Sun Online 2005 Mar 29 [cited on 20 September 2007]. Available at http://modelminority.com/printout1040.html.
45. Wong W. No laughing matter. The Cornell Daily Sun Online 2005 Mar 29 [cited on 20 September 2007]. Available at http://modelminority.com/printout1040.html.
46. Bachman JG, Wallace JM, O'Malley PM, Johnston LD, Kurth CL, Neighbors HW. Racial/ethnic differences in smoking, drinking, and illicit drug use among American high school seniors. Am J Public Health 1991;3:372–377.
47. Wallace JM, Bachman JG. Explaining racial/ethnic differences in adolescent drug use: the impact of background and lifestyle. Soc Probl 1991;38(3):333–357.
48. Appleyard J, Messeri P, Haviland ML. Smoking among Asian American and Hawaiian/Pacific Islander youth: data from the 2000 National Youth Tobacco Survey. Asian Am Pac Isl J Health 2001; 9(1):5–14.
49. Kershaw JM. AAPI youth tobacco use; a comparative analysis of current cigarette use data from the Florida, Texas, and National Youth Tobacco Surveys. Asian Am Pac Isl J Health 2001;9(1):25–33.
50. Glanz K, Maskarinec G, Carlin L. Ethnicity, sense of coherence, and tobacco use among adolescents. Ann Behav Med 2005;29(3):192–199.
51. James WH, Kim GK, Armijo E. The influence of ethnic identity on drug use among ethnic minority adolescents. J Drug Educ 2000;30(3):265–280.
52. Mayeda DT, Hishinuma ES, Nishimura ST, Garcia-Santiago O, Mark GY. Asian/Pacific Islander youth violence prevention center: interpersonal violence and deviant behaviors among youth in Hawaii. J Adolesc Health 2006;39(2):276, e1–e11.
53. Hawaii state and county quickfacts. U.S. Census Bureau Web site [cited 2007 Dec 15]. Available from: URL: http://quickfacts.census.gov/qfd/states/15000.html.
54. Office of minority health and health disparities: Native Hawaiian and other Pacific Islander (NHOPI) populations resource page. Center for Disease Control web site [cited on 15 December 2007]. Available at http://www.cdc.gov/omhd/Populations/NHOPI/NHOPI.htm.
55. Goldberg ME. Truancy and dropout among Cambodian students: results from a comprehensive high school. Soc Work Educ 1999;21(1):49–63.
56. Fujino DC. The rates, patterns and reasons for forming heterosexual interracial dating relationships among Asian Americans. J Soc Pers Relat 1997;14:809–828.
57. King RB, Harris KM. Romantic relationships among immigrant adolescents. Int Migr Rev 2007; 41(2):344–370.
58. Kodama CM, McEwen MK, Liang CTH, Lee S. A theoretical examination of psychosocial issues for Asian Pacific American students. NASPA J 2001;38(4):411–437.
59. Chung YB, Katayama M. Ethnic and sexual identity development of Asian American lesbian and gay adolescents. In:Ng, KS, editor. Counseling Asian families from a systems perspective. Alexandria, VA: American Counseling Association; 1999, p. 159–169.
60. Masequesmay G. Building allies: linking race, class, gender, and sexuality in Asian American studies. In: Chen EW, Omatsu G, editors. Teaching about Asian Pacific Americans: effective activities, strategies, and assignments for classrooms and communities. Lanham, MD: Rowman & Littlefield Publishers, Inc.; 2006, pp. 57–74.
61. Catalano RF, Berglund ML, Ryan JAM, Lonczak HS, Hawkins JD. Positive youth development in the United States: research findings on evaluations of positive youth development programs. Prev Treat 2002;5(15) [cited on 23 September 2005]. Available at http://journals.apa.org/prevention/volume5/pre0050015a.html.
62. Guerrero APS, Hishinuma ES, Andrade NN, Nishimura ST, Cunanan VL. Correlations among socioeconomic and family factors and academic, behavioral, and emotional difficulties in Filipino adolescents in Hawaii. Int J Soc Psychiatry 2006;52(4):343–359.

63. Oppedal B, Røysamb E, Heyerdahl S. Ethnic group, acculturation, and psychiatric problems in young immigrants. J Child Psychol Psychiatry 2005;46(6):646–660.
64. Bjorck JP, Cuthbertson W, Thurman JW, Yee YS. Ethnicity, coping, and distress among Korean Americans, Filipino Americans, and Caucasian Americans. J Soc Psychol 2001; 141(4):421–442.
65. Bjorck JP, Lee YS, Cohen LH. Control beliefs and faith as stress moderators for Korean American versus Caucasian American Protestants. Am J Community Psychol 1997;25(1):61–72.

Acculturation and Asian American Elderly

Nhi-Ha Trinh and Iqbal Ahmed

Abstract The "graying" of the United States and its increasing ethnic and racial diversification make understanding the particular acculturation issues facing the Asian American elderly important for the mental health clinician. This population faces multiple acculturation stressors making it vulnerable to depression, anxiety, and suicide. In addition, for Asian American elderly suffering from dementia, acculturation can influence the diagnosis, treatment, and attitudes toward caregiving. Understanding these factors is critical for clinicians taking care of the Asian American elderly.

Keywords Asian American elderly · Depression · Suicide · Caregiving · Acculturation stressors · Intergenerational stressors

Contents

Introduction	168
Acculturation and Mental Health Issues in Asian American Elderly	169
Risk of Depression and Anxiety in Asian American Elderly	169
Risk of Suicide in Asian American Elderly	170
Dementia in Asian American Elderly	172
Epidemiology of Dementia in Asian American Elderly	172
Family Perceptions of Dementia in Asian American Elderly	173
Caregiving for Asian American Elderly	174
Patterns of Caregiving in Asian American Families	174
Future Directions and Clinical Implications	175
References	176

N.-H. Trinh (✉)
Massachusetts General Hospital, Depression Clinical Research Program, Boston MA, USA
e-mail: ntrinh@partners.org

Introduction

The "graying" of the United States and its increasing ethnic and racial diversification make understanding the particular acculturation issues facing the Asian American elderly important for the mental health clinician. According to the 2000 Census, by 2030, about 20% of the total US population is projected to be of age 65 and older [1]. In particular, nearly one-fourth of the older foreign-born population in the United States is from Asia, and the Asian American elderly population grew by 76% from 1990 to 2000. Furthermore, this population is projected to grow by 246% from 2000 to 2025, as compared with 9.2 and 73% growth rates in the corresponding years among the European American elderly population [2]. US life expectancy estimates anticipate increased life expectancy for Asian Americans, with 86.2 years on average for Asian American women and 80.2 years for Asian American men [3]. In addition, while the overall death rate of the US population during the period 2002–2004 was 826.5 per 100,000, the Asian or Pacific Islander death rate was half that, only 460.9 per 100,000 [4]. Within the immigrant Asian American elderly group, however, life expectancy may decline with increasing time spent in the United States. Consistent with the acculturative stress hypothesis, immigrants' risks of depression, disability, and chronic disease morbidity appear to increase with increasing length of residence [5].

These demographic shifts in the population of older adults in the United States have led to an increased awareness of the particular needs of the Asian American elderly. As has been discussed in earlier chapters, the acculturation process is multidimensional, including physical, psychological, financial, spiritual, social, language, and family adjustment. This process can be very stressful for immigrant Asian American elders in the United States because they may have fewer resources, such as income, education, and English proficiency, to assist them in adapting to their new life situation. An additional dilemma is that acculturation can occur at different rates for different individuals. The adaptation of Asian American elderly is affected by a number of factors in their premigration history: their countries of origin, including their specific cultural backgrounds, their socioeconomic status in the country of origin, their prior history of living in a modernized urban versus rural environment, and their reasons for immigration (political, economic, familial). Factors in their new environment also affect their ability to integrate; in particular, Asian American elderly may feel more integrated if there are other immigrants at the place of settlement of similar age and background, or if there are institutions such as churches or social clubs.

Children may have more exposure to American culture through school, and their parents through work; in contrast, if Asian American elderly immigrate at an older age, they may find themselves isolated in their new surroundings. As newcomers who have spent much of their life in a different society, they must cognitively, attitudinally, and behaviorally adapt to the new cultural system.

Even daily life events in a new environment may become stressful [6]. In particular, Asian American elderly face particular challenges as they integrate from an Asian culture to the American culture. The former places an emphasis on the group through filial piety, humility, restraint of emotional expression, and a sense of obligation toward elders; the latter is more individualistic, competitive, achievement-oriented, assertive, and more concerned with mastery over one's environment. Elders may find it difficult to adjust to this "American way of life" in their families; as their children and grandchildren acculturate, cultural discontinuity increases in the home. The differences in acculturation among the different generations can lead to intergenerational conflict. These differences may need to be negotiated within the extended family to restore harmony.

Not only is this a large attitudinal change, but also practical challenges exist with language, financial concerns, and navigation of the rules and regulations of a new culture. Role reversals may occur when children and grandchildren become translators and interpreters of American culture for seniors, or when limitations on financial resources translate into a reversal of authority and power in the family. Given these stressors, this population is quite vulnerable to acculturative stress. However, despite the increasing number of Asian American elderly immigrants and the recognition that mental health clinicians should be sensitive to cross-cultural issues in the elderly, there exists a paucity of research regarding these populations [7]. Nevertheless, this population has particular vulnerabilities relating to their immigrant and acculturation status, which, in turn, affect their mental health. In this chapter, we will examine the effects of acculturation on the mental health of elderly Asian Americans and the clinical implications of acculturation stressors on this group.

Acculturation and Mental Health Issues in Asian American Elderly

Risk of Depression and Anxiety in Asian American Elderly

There is increasing recognition of the role of culture and ethnicity in the risk and protective factors of depression, anxiety, and suicidality. However, very little is known about the risk of depression in the Asian Americans and the Asian American elderly in particular. Asian American and Asian immigrant elderly groups are rarely included in national long-term care data sets in sufficient numbers to ensure meaningful analysis [7]. Two large epidemiologic studies, the Epidemiologic Catchment Area Study and the National Co-morbidity Survey, were unable to estimate with confidence the prevalence of depression in Asian Americans as a whole, and the elderly in particular [8, 9]. The Chinese American Psychiatric Epidemiological Study estimated rates of depression in Chinese Americans in Los Angeles County and found low-to-moderate levels of depressive disorders in this predominantly immigrant group [10]. Using Diagnostic and Statistical Manual, Fourth Edition (DSM-IV)-based criteria or major depression, the 1-year prevalence rate of depression was estimated at about 5% or less among community-dwelling people aged 65 and older [11]. Depressive symptoms or syndromes have been found to be more prevalent, with about 15–20% prevalence for community-dwelling elders [12].

If research on depression in Asian American elders is sparse, there exists even less research on anxiety among older Asian Americans. In two studies of older Japanese American adults, anxiety disorders were not as prevalent as compared with depression, but Japanese American adults conceptualized anxiety similarly to the conceptualization of anxiety found in the DSM-IV [13, 14]. However, there was some overlap between the conceptualization of anxiety and depression. For example, some participants used depressive terms, such as irritability, sleep disturbance, and depression, to describe anxiety. Respondents thought risk factors for anxiety would include not being able to relax, having negative thoughts, and ruminating, which are similar to risk factors for depression. Clearly, additional studies are needed to examine more closely the prevalence and phenomenology of both depression and anxiety for this population.

Depression and anxiety may occur frequently in Asian immigrant elders because they have limited resources in dealing with the multiple losses associated with the process of adaptation, acculturation, and family disruption [15]. A few small sample studies of Asian elders also reported that immigrants who were more acculturated to the host society tended to have better mental health status than those who were less acculturated [16, 17]. In a study examining the role of acculturation of older Korean Americans, those with lower levels of acculturation to mainstream American culture were more at risk for depressive symptoms, even after controlling for socioeconomic status [18]. Another study looked at a sample of six different Asian elderly groups (Chinese, Filipino, Indian, Japanese, Korean, and Vietnamese) and examined the association between acculturation stress and depression [19]. Examining the relationship of acculturation stress specifically on depression, they found that about 40% of the sample was depressed, and that acculturation stress caused by the elders' perception of a cultural gap between themselves and their adult children was associated with high depression levels [19]. Studies on Asian American family support have shown that Asian American elders receive a considerable amount of emotional and practical support from their adult children [20, 21]. In addition, studies on the role of social support of family members and its impact on the psychological well-being of elders have found that higher rates of depression are associated with fewer family contacts and smaller social network [22].

Risk of Suicide in Asian American Elderly

A quarter of all late-life suicides are due to depression [23]. Compared with older European Americans, the rates of suicide overall among Asian Americans are significantly lower. Most studies have assessed only three major ethnic groups, the Chinese, Japanese, and Filipinos, with the overwhelming majority focusing on only the first two [24]. One of the studies examining rates of suicide using the 1990 census found that Asian American elderly had 50% of the suicide rate of European American elderly; among the ethnic minorities, however, Asian American elderly had the highest rates of completed suicide [25]. In addition, rates of suicide by Chinese American women greatly exceeded that of Japanese American and European American women, and that rates of completed suicide by Japanese American women were higher than European American women in the 75- to 84-year age group. The author hypothesized that the high rates of suicide seen in Chinese American women may indicate a cohort effect reflecting tension between traditional gender roles and the American ideal of equality. In addition, for both Chinese and Japanese American women, increased risk of depression and suicide may have been associated with the loss of family cohesion as adult children moved away. Interestingly, rates of completed suicide by older European American men exceeded rates for Chinese and Japanese American men; however, after the age of 85 years, this pattern reversed. Baker hypothesized that the high rates in the oldest age group reflected a cohort that immigrated before 1924, before the repeal of the Oriental Exclusion Acts of the 1880s. As a result, these men came to the United States alone and experienced acculturation stress without family support. These patterns continued to persist; more recent data estimates of completed suicide rates in 2000–2004 showed that female Asian Americans over the age of 65 years had the highest completed suicide rates in comparison with European American, Hispanic American, and African American groups [26]. In contrast, male Asian Americans over the age of 65 years had lower completed suicide rates in comparison with European American and Hispanic American groups, but were higher than African American groups [4].

Another study examining completed suicides in San Francisco from 1987 to 1994 found that Asian American women had lower rates of completed suicide as compared with European American women, except in the age of 85 years and older cohort. In contrast, Asian American males were found to have lower rates of suicide as compared with European American men, except between the age of 75 and 84 years [27]. Hanging was the most common means used to complete suicide by Asian Americans, as compared with the use of firearms by European Americans. To explain the higher rates of suicide in the older Asian Americans, the authors hypothesized that these older immigrants came to the United States without their traditional support systems and were confronted with a new idea that the elderly should not be a burden to their children. This created a conflict with their traditional view of being revered for their old age. To explain the method of suicide, the authors postulated that it reflected a pattern in traditional China where hanging is predominantly used.

Not only are Asian American elderly at risk for suicide but they also have a higher proportion of death and suicidal ideation as compared with other minority elder groups. In one study, using the Paykel suicide questionnaire to probe thoughts about death, suicide, or attempts at suicide, Asian American elderly had the highest proportion of Death Ideation (37.8%) or Suicidal Ideation (11.8%) in comparison with African American, Hispanic American, and European American groups [28]. Taken together, these studies reveal not only that Asian American elderly may have higher rates of depression secondary to acculturation stress but also that they are at higher risk for suicide than other ethnic minority groups.

These findings point to the need for more research to understand intergenerational family relationships. The common denominator underlying these studies is the stress that arises when elderly parents feel distant from their adult children, particularly when the elderly have high expectations of family solidarity and interdependence [15]. The resulting generational split of the family may be both a source and an indicator of intergenerational conflicts. For Asian American elder parents, they may be confronted with the loss of respect, as their role as cultural conservator and family decision maker may be undermined. Interestingly, length of residence in the United States also predicted higher levels of depression in Asian American elders [19]. This finding is reversed from other studies, where increasing length of residence in the United States corresponded to lower levels of depression in Asian American adults younger than 65 years [29]. One hypothesis is that the longer Asian American immigrant elderly have lived in the United States, the more likely they are to have American-born children and grandchildren. Their descendents' acculturation and family expectations differ from their parents and grandparents [30]. This heightened cultural gap between the generations may cause elders' anxiety regarding their role in the family and may increase their risk for depression, hopelessness, and risk for suicide.

Dementia in Asian American Elderly

Epidemiology of Dementia in Asian American Elderly

Researchers have observed ethnic and cross-national differences in the frequency of different types of dementia. Dementia is characterized by a decline in memory and other cognitive abilities, ultimately interfering with daily, social, and occupational functioning. In general, overall rates of dementia are similar cross-nationally and cross-culturally, but notable differences exist in rates of dementia subtypes [31]. Although some Asian American elders such as the Chinese and Japanese have a higher risk of developing vascular dementia as compared with Alzheimer dementia in their homeland, data suggest that the influence of acculturation modifies their risk of developing Alzheimer dementia. The Ni Hon-San study of Japanese migration from Japan to Honolulu suggests that as migrating Japanese groups become more acculturated to the United States, rates of vascular dementia decline and rates of Alzheimer dementia increase to be more similar to rates in the European American population in the United States. This finding suggests a cultural and environmental influence on the development of dementia [32]. The authors postulate that lower rates of vascular dementia may be secondary to improved control over environmental risk factors, such as a change in diet or improved control over hypertension as Japanese American elderly acculturated. Although the exact mechanism remains to be clarified, it is clear that as certain Asian American groups acculturate into the United States, new patterns of the prevalence of dementia emerge.

Finally, although similar rates of dementia exist for Asian American elderly as for other groups in the United States, individual characteristics among Asian American elderly can create barriers in the diagnosis of dementia. Among older Asian populations, language differences are among the most common reasons for the avoidance of health-care services by community members as well as errors in diagnosis by clinicians [33]. Not only do language barriers make diagnosis dementia difficult, only 32% of Asian American elders have 8 years or less of formal education, making screening instruments for dementia difficult to interpret [34]. These obstacles combined with Asian American family perceptions of dementia make it difficult for Asian American elderly to seek out help and receive treatment.

Family Perceptions of Dementia in Asian American Elderly

Caregivers of Asian American elderly may have an understanding of dementia that reflects more traditional views of aging. In a study of adult family caregivers, Asian American caregivers were the most likely to adhere to "folk models" of dementia, which attribute dementia-related changes as a result of psychosocial stress in combination with "normal" aging processes [35]. This difference in the family's perception of the etiology of the illness may influence the time to presentation to medical and psychiatric care. In addition, the family may not recognize their ailing relative's difficulties. In a study of Japanese elderly, family members failed to notice problems with memory, and the majority of subjects with dementia had not received medical evaluation for their illness [36]. Lack of access to education regarding the characteristics of dementia was a main factor influencing their inability to recognize dementia in their elderly relatives. In addition, out of respect for their elderly relatives, family members reported trying to ignore memory difficulties to "save face" for their elderly relatives. The idea that caregivers would not seek outside support and interventions out of respect for and duty toward elders is a theme that recurs in other interviews with Asian American caregivers [37]. For Asian American families, dementia may be a mental health diagnosis with which they may have an incomplete understanding. As with many mental health issues, dementia symptoms may carry a great deal of shame, preventing Asian American families from seeking intervention and treatment for their elders.

Caregiving for Asian American Elderly

Patterns of Caregiving in Asian American Families

In the United States, 18% of Asian Americans provide informal care for their elderly family members, as compared with 21% of European Americans and African Americans and 16% of Latino Americans [38]. In addition, in many Asian American cultures, the son's family traditionally has the most responsibility for taking care of the older parent. Given traditional gender roles, the burden of daily care falls on the oldest son's wife; this is in contrast to the mainstream US populations, where the spouse is the first-choice provider, followed by daughters [39]. These values come from a collectivist approach, which emphasizes the welfare of the extended family versus a Western individualist way of thinking [40]. Also underlying this strong preference is an emphasis on filial piety, or the belief that each individual has an obligation to older generations [41]. As a result, there is a strong preference for family caregiving versus institutionalized care. In a survey of Japanese American and European American elders, Japanese Americans were more likely to rely on loved ones than European Americans, who were more likely to rely on paid providers [42].

However, although Asian Americans rely on their families, this causes a significant burden on caregivers. Studies of caregivers of Asian American elderly have shown that, as compared with European American caregivers, Asian American caregivers are engaged in significantly higher numbers of caregiving tasks, and report lower levels of use of formal support. Asian American caregivers also reported a lower quality of relationship with the care recipient, and were more likely to use emotion-focused coping. In this type of coping, caregivers try to deal with their stress by eliminating unpleasant emotions by denial, wishful thinking, or rethinking the emotion in a positive way through relaxation. In contrast, caregivers, using problem-focused coping, take action to modify the underlying stressful situation. As a result, Asian American caregivers had higher levels of depression, did not feel satisfied from caregiving, and had poorer physical health as compared with European American caregivers [43]. In a study of Korean American caregivers, these caregivers felt a higher degree of caregiving burden and lower levels of emotional and practical support as compared with European American caregivers [39]. Researchers from these studies hypothesized that Asian American caregivers, largely daughters-in-law or daughters bound by a sense of obligation and respect for their elders, may find themselves in stressful roles vis-à-vis their elderly relatives. As Asian American elderly continue to expect that their children will take care of them, the younger generation will find themselves conflicted between their sense of duty to their extended family and the adoption of American values that focus on individuality and the nuclear family. Placing their elderly relatives in a nursing home may not feel like an option to this generation; they may find themselves "sandwiched" between the expectations of taking care of their elders with having to take care of their own families. Combined with the practicalities of caregiving, this may result in a higher degree of caregiving burden, and eventually, caregiver burnout.

Future Directions and Clinical Implications

Ultimately, more research is needed on the prevalence of anxiety and depression among older Asian Americans. In addition, much research to date has focused on East Asian groups, such as the Korean, Japanese, and Chinese, and little is known about Southeast Asian and South Asian elderly groups. Given the unique characteristics of each group with regard to language abilities, educational level, and generational and immigration status, researchers may consider expanding their attention to include other specific ethnic groups in the future.

Multiple practical and cultural barriers to care exist for Asian American elderly. For the Asian American elderly and their families, these include limited knowledge about available services, which may not be sensitive to cultural needs. They also suffer from a lack of financial resources and access to transportation. Finally, cultural norms may play a role, including a strong belief and preference for family care. In the Family Caregiving in the US survey, Asian American caregivers identified numerous barriers to getting supportive services for their elderly care recipients. Reasons for not being able to get appropriate services for their elders include issues with service unavailability, cost and eligibility, personal feelings of guilt for not fulfilling family obligations, and pride in self-sufficiency [44]. Researchers must better understand help-seeking patterns of older Asian American adults and their families, examine who they turn to for assistance and support, and evaluate the types of services that are provided to those who seek help.

Effective culturally appropriate prevention and treatment strategies must be developed that incorporate services geared to meet specific needs of Asian American elders and their caregivers. We must consider developing services in Asian languages, and incorporating cultural values such as respect for elders and cooperation in our interventions. In addition, we must consider providing social support for caregivers, making available information regarding diagnoses of mental health disorders and community resources, and developing initiatives to screen for dementia and depression in primary care offices and community centers. As the Asian American elderly population grows in the twenty-first century, increasing the availability of culturally competent formal services such as nursing homes or assisted living will be critical.

In the meantime, understanding the particular dilemmas that Asian American elderly face will enable clinicians to better serve this population. Awareness of the individual's particular sociocultural background, acculturation stressors, and expectations for aging will enable clinicians to better engage with their Asian American elderly patients and their families. The knowledge that mental health issues are prevalent and yet underrecognized for this population must prompt us to renew our efforts to reach out to this underserved population at risk.

References

1. Hetzel L and Smith A. The 65 years and over population: 2000. Census 2000 Brief, Washington DC, 2001. Accessed on March 17, 2007 at http://www.census.gov/prod/2001pubs/c2kbr01-10.pdf.
2. Census of Population: Asian and Pacific Islanders in the United States. US Census Bureau, Washington DC, 1990. Accessed on March 17, 2007 at http://www.census.gov/prod/cen1990/cp3/cp-3-5.pdf
3. Manton KG. Longevity and long-lived populations. In: Birren JE, ed. Encyclopedia of gerontology: Age, aging, and the aged. San Diego, Academic Press, 1996: 83–95.
4. Health, United States 2006. Center for Disease Control, Atlanta, 2006. Accessed on March 17, 2007 at http://www.cdc.gov/nchs/data/hus/hus06.pdf#summary
5. Singh GK and Miller BA. Health, life expectancy, and mortality patterns among immigrant populations in the United States. Canadian Journal of Public Health 2004; 95(3): 14–21.
6. Kalavar JM and Willigen JV. Older Asian Indians resettled in America: Narratives about households, culture and generation. Journal of Cross-Cultural Gerontology 2005; 20: 213–230.
7. Mui AC and Kang SY. Acculturation stress and depression among Asian immigrant elders. Social Work 2006; 51(3): 243–255.
8. Zhang AY and Snowden LR. Ethnic characteristics of mental disorders in five US communities. Cultural Diversity and Ethnic Minority Psychology 1999; 5(2): 134–146.
9. Blazer DG, Kessler RC, McGonagle KA and Swartz MS. The prevalence and distribution of major depression in a national community sample: The National Comorbidity Survey. The American Journal of Psychiatry 1994; 151(7): 979–986.
10. Takeuchi DT, Chung RC, Lin KM et al. Lifetime and twelve-month prevalence rates of major depressive episodes and dysthymia among Chinese Americans in Los Angeles. The American Journal of Psychiatry 1998; 155(10): 1407–1414.
11. Mui AC, Burnette D and Chen LM. Cross-cultural assessment of geriatric depression: A review of the CES-D and the GDS. Journal of Mental Health and Aging 2001; 7(1): 137–164.
12. Gallo JJ and Lebowitz BF. The epidemiology of common late-life mental disorders in the community: Themes for a new century. Psychiatric Services 1999; 50: 1158–1166.
13. Yamamoto J, Machiaawa S, Araki F et al. Mental health of elderly Asian Americans in Los Angeles. The American Journal of Social Psychiatry 1985; 5: 37–46.
14. Iwamasa GY, Hilliard KM and Osata SM. Conceptualizing anxiety and depression: The older Japanese American adults perspective. Clinical Gerontologist 1998; 19: 13–26.
15. Mui AC. Depression among elderly Chinese immigrants: An exploratory study. Social Work 1996; 41: 633–645.
16. Pang KYC. Symptoms of depression in elderly Korean immigrants: Narration and the healing process. Culture, Medicine and Psychiatry 1998; 22: 93–122.
17. Stokes SC, Thompson LW, Murphy S, and Gallagher-Thompson D. Screening for depression in immigrant Chinese-American elders: Results of a pilot study. Journal of Gerontological Social Work 2001; 36(1/2): 27–44.
18. Jang Y, Kim G and Chiriboga D. Acculturation and manifestation of depressive symptoms among Korean American older adults. Aging and Mental Health 2005; 9(6): 500–507.

19. Mui AC and Kang SY. Acculturation stress and depression among Asian immigrant elders. Social Work 2006; 51(3): 243–255.
20. Mui AC. Stress, coping and depression among elderly Korean immigrants. Journal of Human Behavior in the Social Environment 2001; 3(3/4), 281–299.
21. Shibusawa T and Mui AC. Stress, coping, and depression among Japanese American elders. Journal of Gerontological Social Work 2001; 36(1/2): 63–81.
22. Lee MS, Crittenden KS and Yu E. Social support and depression among elderly Korean immigrants in the United States. International Journal of Aging and Human Development 1996; 42: 313–327.
23. American Association of Retired Persons (AARP). Depression in later life. Washington DC: American Association of Retired Persons, 1997.
24. Leong FTL, Leach MM, Yeh C and Chou E. Suicide among Asian Americans: What do we know? What do we need to know? Death Studies, 2007; 31(5): 417–434.
25. Baker FM. Suicide among ethnic minority elderly: A statistical and psychosocial perspective. Journal of Geriatric Psychiatry 1994; 27: 241–264.
26. McKenzie K, Serfaty M, and Crawford M. Suicide in ethnic minority groups. British Journal of Psychiatry 2003; 183: 100–101.
27. Shiang, J., Blinn, R., Bongar, B., Stephens, B., Allison, D., and Schatzberg, A. Suicide in San Francisco, CA: A comparison of Caucasian and Asian groups: 1987–1994. Suicide and Life-Threatening Behavior 1997; 27(1): 80–91.
28. Bartels SJ, Coakley E, Oxman TE et al. Suicide and death ideation in older primary care patients with depression, anxiety, and at-risk alcohol use. American Journal of Geriatric Psychiatry 2002; 10(4): 417–427.
29. Mills TL and Henretta JC. Racial, ethnic and sociodemographic differences in the level of psychosocial distress among older Americans. Research on Aging, 2007; 23(2): 131–152.
30. Diego AT, Yamamoto J, Nguyen LH, and Hifumi SS. Suicide in the elderly: Profiles of Asians and Whites. Asian American and Pacific Islander Journal of Health 1994; 2:49–57.
31. Watari K and Gatz M. Dementia: A cross-cultural perspective on risk Factors. Generations 2002; Spring: 32–38.
32. Graves AB, Larson EB, White LR, Teng EL and Homma A. Opportunities and challenges in international collaborative epidemiologic research of dementia and its subtypes: Studies between Japan and the U.S. International Psychogeriatrics 1994; 6: 209–223.
33. Gilman SC, Justice J and Saepharn K et al. Use of traditional and modern health services by Laotian refugees. Western Journal of Medicine 1992; 157: 310–315.
34. Espino DV and Lewis R. Dementia in older minority populations: Issues of prevalence, diagnosis, and treatment. American Journal of Geriatric Psychiatry 1998; 6: S19–S25.
35. Hinton L, Franz C, Yeo G and Levkoff S. Conceptions of dementia in a multiethnic sample of family caregivers. JAGS 2005; 53: 1405–1410.
36. Ross GW, Abbott RD, Petrovitch H et al. Frequency and characteristics of silent dementia among elderly Japanese-American men. The Honolulu-Asia Aging Study. JAMA 1997; 277(10): 800–805.
37. Dilworth-Anderson P and Gibson BE. The cultural influence of values, norms, meanings, and perceptions in understanding dementia in ethnic minorities. Alzheimer Disease and Associated Disorders 2002; 16(2): S56–S63.
38. National Alliance for Caregiving (NAC) and the American Association of Retired Persons (AARP). Family caregiving in the US: Findings from a national survey. Washington DC: NAC, AARP, 1997.
39. Youn G, Knight BG, Jeong HS and Benton D. Difference in familism values and caregiving outcomes among Korean, Korean American and White American dementia caregivers. Psychology and Aging 1999; 14(3): 355–364.
40. Segall MH, Lonner WJ, and Berry JW. Cross-cultural psychology as a scholarly discipline: On the flowering of culture in behavior research. American Psychologist 1998; 53: 1101–1110.

41. Sung K. Motivations for parent care: The case of filial children in Korea. International Journal of Aging and Human Development 1992; 34: 109–124.
42. Young HM, McCormick WM and Vitaliano PP. Attitudes toward community-based services among Japanese-American Families, The Gerontologist 2002; 42(6): 814–825.
43. Pinquart M and Sorensen S. Ethnic differences in stressors, resources, and psychological outcomes of family caregiving: A meta-analysis. The Gerontologist 2005; 45(1): 90–106.
44. Li H. Barriers to and unmet needs for supportive services: Experiences of Asian-American Caregivers. Journal of Cross-Cultural Gerontology 2004; 19:241–260.

Clinical Insights from Working with Immigrant Asian Americans and Their Families: Focus on Acculturation Stressors

Nalini V. Juthani and A.S. Mishra

Abstract Using five clinical cases, this chapter discusses particular clinical dilemmas faced when working with Asian American immigrants. Topics discussed through the five cases include the following: (1) Intra- and Intergenerational acculturative familial conflicts; (2) Acculturation factors relevant to the onset of panic disorder; (3) Somatization, stigma, acculturative differences between patient and clinician; (4) Alcoholism, domestic violence, and intra-generational conflict; and (5) Acculturation considerations in the recognition and treatment of serious psychiatric illness. In addition, the authors address specific clinical challenges and recommendations based on gender and age.

Keywords Asian American mental health · Intragenerational conflict · Intergenerational conflict · Acculturation · Mental illness stigmatization

Contents

Case 1: Case of Conflict Secondary to Intra- and Intergenerational Acculturation	180
Background and Description of Stressors	180
The Case of Mr. and Mrs. S	181
Summary	183
Case 2: Case of Generalized Anxiety and Panic Attacks: Recent Acculturation Stressors	183
Background and Description of Stressors	183
The Case of Mr. P	184
Summary	185
Case 3: Case of Somatization and of Attitudes Toward Mental Health Treatment Based on the Degree of Acculturation	186
Background and Description of Stressors	186
The Case of Mrs. D	187
Summary	188

N.V. Juthani (✉)
Scarsdale, NY, USA
e-mail: nalini.juthani@gmail.com

Case 4: Case of Alcoholism, Domestic Violence, and Intragenerational Stress 188
   Background and Description of Stressors 188
   The Case of Mr. and Mrs. B 189
   Summary 190
Case 5: Case of the Stigma of Major Mental Illness 190
   Background and Description of Stressors 190
   Case of Mrs. T 191
   Summary 192
Implications for Practice: Specific Subcategories 193
Treatment: Special Considerations for Psychopharmacological Management 195
Conclusion 196
References 196

The culturally astute clinician will remain alert to the differences among individual patients and families from any given subculture and will be on guard against stereotyping. Clinicians must ensure that generalizations do not become stereotypes used to define individual patients. One needs to distinguish a *cultural hypothesis* from a *cultural stereotype* because prior familiarity with a particular culture may lead to inaccurate assumptions. For example, a cultural stereotype is the belief that all immigrants are inflexibly frozen in time after immigration to the United States. A clinician working with a cultural hypothesis would use this stereotype as just a hypothesis, to be verified for each individual under treatment. The concepts presented in this chapter are intended to serve as guides (cultural hypotheses) rather than as a rigid list of cultural attributes (cultural stereotypes). We will highlight the cultural hypotheses and stereotypes in the clinical scenarios that follow and hope to add a clinical dimension to the many take-home points mentioned previously in this book. To protect patient confidentiality, the following cases do not represent actual patients and are instead fictionalized composites of several cases.

Case 1: Case of Conflict Secondary to Intra- and Intergenerational Acculturation

Background and Description of Stressors

With immigration comes a clash of cultures, and after the clash, new identities may emerge. Often within the same family, individual family members may emerge from the acculturation process with different identities and present as (a) hyper identified, (b) overidentified/more assimilated, (c) more equally bicultural, or (d) more marginalized. *Hyper identification* occurs when one becomes more traditional than one was before migration. *Over identification* occurs through assimilation, when one becomes more Americanized and disregards one's native culture. *Bicultural identification* occurs when one is able to develop a new identity by integrating the values from both the host and the culture of origin. Finally, *marginalization* occurs when one is not only more traditional than one was before migration but also retreats from the mainstream of society. [1, 2] These variations in the degree of acculturation frequently lead to intrafamilial and intergenerational conflicts in the immediate aftermath of migration or may appear years after the initial migration.

The Case of Mr. and Mrs. S

Mr. S was a successful businessman in Korea. While in their forties, he and his wife migrated to the United States on a business visa. Mr. S struggled to be accepted in the business world in this country. He was frustrated and angry. Eventually, he decided to start a self-operated business in which his wife and children were all expected to work at different shifts so that he did not have to pay hired help. This was a major change in the lifestyle of this family. In this self-employed business, he and his family had to do all the chores from cleaning to selling goods. From his hierarchical cultural way of thinking, this was an insult. Culturally, it was important for him to tell his extended family and friends in their home country that he was a successful businessman in America. Obviously, he and his wife could not share the truth of his current situation with the extended family back home.

Eventually, he began to do well in his business. He also started to take on more "American" ways, dressing more "American," communicating in English with his family, and changing his manner of verbal and nonverbal communication. In addition, he began to use "American" English slang, which is looked down upon in Korea. On the other hand, his wife, a rather traditional woman who had never worked outside the house in Korea, began to feel isolated and overworked. She did not have the support systems she had back home. Gradually, she began to drift from her husband, who was changing too rapidly for her to comprehend. She began to cope by clinging to her three children, overprotecting them, and demanding they observe the cultural values with which she had grown up. She did not allow them to play with the other children on their block. They were neither allowed to bring home other American school children nor allowed to have any play dates. The children were obligated to work in the family's business after completing their homework. Mrs. S believed in attending church weekly and forced her husband and children to accompany her.

Within a couple of years after immigration, Mr. S had become a different man. He wanted to eat fast food every night, and his wife felt that he rejected the Korean food she had historically cooked for the family. She perceived this behavior as a rejection of her and felt he was "becoming too Americanized," a term used to describe unacceptable behavior(s) within their cultural norms. She adapted by becoming even more involved in the Korean church and limited herself to socializing only with other Korean women.

Her son, the oldest child, was very obedient initially at the time of immigration. When he was argumentative with her, she perceived him as "rebelling" against her. This behavior is considered to be disrespectful and disobedient in Korean culture. He was conflicted between his own desires to enjoy American culture and his worries that he would offend his mother. He coped by trying to act "American" outside the home and by acting more "Korean" inside the home. It took him a long time to strike a balance and develop his own emerging identity. He began to excel in school and earned academic awards that brought honor to his family. He developed friendships with classmates from a variety of cultures. He played sports of all kinds, worked in the store a couple of hours on the weekends, and spoke both languages: English outside the home and the Korean dialect his mother spoke with him at home. He felt comfortable eating food from all cultures when he went out with his friends, but unlike his father, he enjoyed his mother's home-cooked meals as well. The two younger girls, however, continued to follow their mother and became increasingly isolated.

Family discord began to occur slowly but steadily and reached its height when the son decided to go to an Ivy League college away from home. During this time, his father was spending less and less time at home. He socialized with "the guys" in the evenings after closing his store. He did not react strongly against his son's decision. However, he did feel strongly that such decisions are not to be made by a son without the permission of his father. His mother was shocked to hear her son's announcement. She wondered, "How can he dare to take such a major step in his life without consulting his father and mother?" She felt increasingly isolated, lonely, and betrayed and would cry often. She felt rejected by her son. She did not express her emotions to anyone and became withdrawn, not eating much, and lost all interest in cooking for the family. She talked about her difficulties with her local priest, who offered some advice and wanted to speak to the family. However, her husband and son refused to meet the priest. A European American friend suggested that Mr. S seek professional help for his wife. Only a Korean American family friend, who had been in the United States for 20 years, was able to convince the family to meet a Korean American mental health clinician from the same cultural background as the family. Mrs. S and her family agreed to this suggestion.

A male clinician was consulted. He identified the following cultural adaptations/identities of each of these family members: *hyper identification* characterized Mrs. S, *overidentification* was Mr. S's adaptation, and the oldest son was *bicultural*. Many common issues were addressed. For example, some Asian patients like Mrs. S, may prefer being cared for by a clinician from their own culture because of the language and cultural connection. Her treatment helped her family pay attention to her feelings of loneliness and rejection by her husband and son. The male clinician was able to relate well with the two male figures in the family of Mrs. S. The clinician involved the entire family in the treatment. In this case, this was relevant because Asian culture emphasizes and values family involvement and group decision-making, and because Mrs. S. stated this as a preference.

Summary

1. The clinician in this case helped the entire family to reframe the son's choice of an Ivy League college in a more culturally acceptable way. He helped them to see the son's accomplishment as bringing honor to the entire family and not as a disobedient act. In addition, he helped them to consider that going to an out-of-state college was a sacrifice that the entire family would be making to achieve this honor. The entire family, including Mrs. S, was then able to accept the son's going away to study as a sacrifice rather than as an act to fulfill an individual's desire.
2. This case demonstrates that a broad spectrum of acculturation of the individual members of a family, ranging from traditional to more Western, may be seen in the same family. One must not assume that complete acculturation occurs in individuals who have lived in this country for several decades or even generations.

Case 2: Case of Generalized Anxiety and Panic Attacks: Recent Acculturation Stressors

Background and Description of Stressors

Stress arises when a person's ability to cope with many changes over a short period of time is taxed. This stress is evident even when the changes are pleasant such as marriage, moving into a new home, or having a new baby. Clearly, Asian immigrants experience numerous changes in their lives. For example, upon arrival in the United States, new immigrants have to adjust to a new and unfamiliar environment. If English is a second language, their first language can affect their accent, intonation, vocabulary, syntax, and use of idiomatic expressions in English. As a result, their English may not sound like native-born Americans. This may cause embarrassment while talking to other Americans. Also, Asian American immigrants who do not have higher degrees (and some that do) may end up in low-paying jobs. Consequently, many find little reward or fulfillment in their work and experience a sharp decline in their socioeconomic status and life style. In addition, Asian Americans experience more ambiguity in nonfamilial social relationships. They may not feel acquainted with Western social customs and social interactions, and thus may have more difficulty making new friends, further reducing their support system. All of these factors account for increased levels of anxiety among Asian immigrants [3, 4].

Add to this the possibility of traumatization either pre- or postmigration, such patients can present with generalized anxiety, panic attacks, phobias, and posttraumatic stress disorder (PTSD).

The Case of Mr. P

Mr. P was a 38-year-old male who had emigrated from India after receiving his engineering degree. He was single, from a "well-to-do" family, with a well-paying job. A family friend suggested to his father that engineers had better opportunities in America. Mr. P had always lived at home and commuted from home throughout his college years. Although reluctant to travel so far away from home, pressured by his father, he decided to pursue his career in the United States.

Mr. P was able to overcome some initial struggles such as finding a job, cooking for himself, and learning new ways of life in an unfamiliar environment. However, he lived a rather lonely and isolated life because he could not find "appropriate" friends with the educational status and background of which his family would approve. He missed the familiarity of home, convenience of having servants, and a family setting where his needs were taken care of by others. He was anxious every time he had to face a new challenge. He no longer had his familiar supportive network and became anxious and worried.

Mr. P lived in a one-bedroom apartment in an urban center. One day, coming home from work, he was assaulted by a group of teenagers. He lost his wallet, watch, and a very important gold necklace that his mother had put around his neck when he left home to come to the United States. "This necklace is a religious symbol which will always protect you," his mother said with her good byes to her son. Mr. P had not taken this necklace off since leaving home, and would hold the necklace in his hand and pray when he felt very anxious. Now this precious coping strategy had been stolen from him.

Mr. P was tremulous and shaken up emotionally by the assault. He was grateful that he was not physically hurt and escaped with a few bruises, but he felt he could not talk to anyone. He was too scared to inform the police and did not want to call his parents for fear that they would worry. When he realized that the necklace his mother had given him was stolen, he began to feel vulnerable and fearful all the time. He watched his back and took all the protective measures he could when commuting. He began to feel increasingly anxious while going to work and took frequent sick days.

One day at work, he developed shortness of breath, shaking, palpitations, and felt he was going to pass out. His boss took him to the emergency room. The diagnostic work-up yielded no concerning medical conditions. A psychiatric consultant in the emergency room diagnosed him with panic attacks. These attacks recurred several times in the subsequent months. Mr. P continued to see different doctors in the emergency room setting, and each time, he was prescribed benzodiazepines that he did not take. He considered returning back home to his parents. At this point, he told his family what was happening, and his father traveled to the United States to take care of him. Prior to leaving, his father consulted his family physician in India. This family doctor advised him that his son may need to see a psychiatrist. Upset with this news, the father declared, "My son is not crazy! Also, I have to think about getting him a wife!" Of note, typically in India, diagnosed psychiatric illness precludes the chances of finding an appropriate marital partner. The family physician convinced him to get him psychiatric treatment in the United States, reassuring the father that no one need find out about it in the home country.

A South Asian psychiatrist from the same background was consulted. The psychiatrist identified a number of culturally relevant stressors and factors during the initial evaluation. Concerned for the patient's history of nonadherence, the psychiatrist prescribed a short course of benzodiazepines and addressed this with the patient as she outlined the treatment plan and provided psychoeducation about the nature and course of treatment. The psychiatrist also tried to explore and understand his early upbringing, but the patient thought it was totally irrelevant to his suffering. The psychiatrist was able to recognize that exploratory therapy was culturally unacceptable to the patient. The patient and his father wanted the doctor to take the role of an advisor and teacher. Responding to their concerns, the psychiatrist prescribed cognitive behavioral therapy. Mr. P learned relaxation therapy and continued to follow the treatment regimen, eventually giving him relief from his anxiety symptoms.

Summary

1. The clinician communicated respect for the family and the cultural values they held dear. She showed respect for the patient's belief system, for his religion, and his faith in religious symbols. She took a detailed immigration history to understand relevant stressors as well as how the patient had coped with stress.
2. The clinician took an active role in educating the patient. She reviewed with the patient some of the healthier ways of coping in an unfamiliar environment. She used cognitive behavioral therapy to help him cope with his anxiety. She reassured the patient that the medications would be needed for a short period of time, which helped with treatment adherence.
3. The clinician explored the patient's faith in meditation and gave him permission to utilize alternative treatments. As a result, the patient felt that he could be honest with his doctor, trust her more, and work with her to overcome his suffering.
4. The patient's father was included in the treatment with the patient's consent. The psychiatrist was aware that confidentiality issues are understood differently in Asian cultures and family involvement may be expected.

5. The psychiatrist's sensitivity to culturally valued issues such as interdependence versus independence, hierarchical organization, and spiritual beliefs of the family was effective in her work with the patient.

Case 3: Case of Somatization and of Attitudes Toward Mental Health Treatment Based on the Degree of Acculturation

Background and Description of Stressors

Many Asian American immigrants somatize their psychological suffering. Their psychological distress often manifests as physical complaints such as chronic headaches, digestive troubles, vague aches and pains, and insomnia. For example, the language for "depression" does not exist in many cultures. When the tongue does not do the talking, the body does, leaving depression to masquerade as a psychosomatic illness. It may present as a multiplicity of symptoms: lack of energy, headache, chronic fatigue, aches and pains, chest pain, gastrointestinal symptoms, skin allergies, rash, intractable itching, leucorrhea, hysterical seizures, blindness, and fugue states. These symptoms can lead to substance abuse, domestic violence, decreased effectiveness at work/school, irritability, social isolation, impaired relationships, controlling behaviors, insecurities, self-doubt, and extreme possessiveness [5].

Clinicians and researchers have identified several possibilities to understand this somatization. Immigrants may come from cultures that discourage direct emotional expression and instead favor somatic expression of psychic distress [6]. The mind–body dichotomy that is so prevalent in the Western conceptualization of disease process and symptom formation is rarely encountered in the Asian culture. In some Asian cultures, emotions are attributed to various body organs, like the heart, liver, brain, gut, spleen, and even blood.

Thus, Asian immigrants may culturally express their distress in ways that are acceptable and not stigmatized within their native culture. By reporting physical complaints, they may seek medical treatment without having to face the shame that is usually associated with reporting purely psychological problems. They tend to understand psychological problems as "character weakness." In addition, Asian American immigrants may resort to their traditional herbal and alternative treatments prior to consulting a family physician. Because they tend to believe that psychiatric treatment is provided to "crazy" people, they are more likely to consult a family or general physician for somatic symptoms and expect short-term pharmacological treatment. Asian American immigrants may have very limited knowledge of how psychotherapy works and view it as a Western concept.

The Case of Mrs. D

Mrs. D, a recent immigrant from Pakistan, sought treatment for chronic headaches, insomnia, and vague body aches and pains. She told her family physician that she sought treatment intermittently from different general physicians whenever these symptoms worsened; however, no one could cure her problems. Her Pakistani friend accompanied her to the appointment and told the physician that even herbal treatment had failed. The physician inquired about some of these alternative treatment modalities as well as some of the symptoms of depression, which he noted were present. The physician discovered that the patient had immigrated with her husband to the United States about 4 years ago to seek a better economic life. Family history revealed that her husband drank alcohol of which she did not approve. Her extended family back home was upset that she did not yet have children. She took menial part-time jobs to supplement her husband's salary, which was not adequate to support having children.

The physician performed a basic workup and some blood tests, all of which came back within normal limits. He referred the patient to a psychiatrist. The patient vehemently protested that she was not "crazy," no one in her family was crazy, and that she would never do something that would bring shame to the family whether in the United States or back home. Reluctantly, she added that she did not have money to pay for such treatment. She felt that the physician had betrayed her trust and rejected her by referring her to a psychiatrist. When the physician understood her discomfort, he referred her to a social worker from a South Asian background, which the patient accepted.

The social worker explored her physical symptoms and identified them as an expression of her suffering. She explained the mind–body–spirit connection to the patient, which was more culturally acceptable. The social worker encouraged the patient to express her difficulties of being in a new culture and in a new country where she felt isolated from her supports. Over a period of time, the patient conveyed her difficulties about her husband, who continued to drink alcohol excessively. She was able to express fear that her husband would be fired from his job and leave them with no income. In the sessions with her social worker, she was able to express her anger toward him and toward her extended family members, who were nagging her to have children. The patient remained afraid to have children as long as she felt economically insecure. She cried intermittently in the sessions with the social worker, and stated that she had been having more crying episodes and lacked interest in daily activities. With her social worker's encouragement, the patient was then referred to a psychiatrist while the social worker remained as the primary clinician.

Summary

1. The clinician recognized that the tendency to somatize psychological problems was a way to express emotional distress. She was able to highlight and validate the mind–body–spirit connection to the patient.
2. The social worker was a less-threatening clinician for the patient and less stigmatizing compared with a psychiatrist. The patient felt less shame and feared less-negative social consequence in seeking her help.
3. The social worker accepted the patient's belief in alternative treatments and encouraged the patient to try medical treatment with a psychiatrist while remaining as the primary member of the treatment team.
4. This team approach to treatment, consisting of a primary care physician, who addressed the patient's medical concerns, a social worker, and eventually a psychiatrist, carried less stigma for this patient. In cases like these, clinical teams working collaboratively and longitudinally will help the patient develop a therapeutic alliance and become more comfortable with psychiatric treatment.

Case 4: Case of Alcoholism, Domestic Violence, and Intragenerational Stress

Background and Description of Stressors

Asian Americans view substance abuse, especially alcoholism, as a medical as well as a behavioral problem needing moral treatment to rebuild character [7]. Immigrants often face conflicts between the values of the home culture and the host culture. They face these issues in day-to-day interactions with mainstream society both at work and at home. These cultural conflicts can lead to anger, fearfulness, anxiety, depression, loss of self-esteem, a loss of sense of self, as well as substance abuse.

Often, in their countries of origin, Asian immigrants, when faced with conflicts, reach out to extended family and wise men or women in their community. Many may not have similar supportive networks in their new land. If they could reach out to their new communities, these conflicts may be alleviated and not lead to severe consequences. Unfortunately, many immigrant families are socially isolated. To further compound their isolation, immigrants often work two to three jobs to support their families in the United States and may be supporting extended families at home. They do not have the time and resources to develop new supportive networks in the host country. Thus, this unavailability of family and community support in times of crises can make them vulnerable to social risk factors such as alcoholism, drug abuse, antisocial behavior, and domestic violence.

The Case of Mr. and Mrs. B

Mr. and Mrs. B arrived in the United States from the Philippines with high hopes of making a good living. They were both professionals. After arriving, they learned that to apply for a license to practice medicine they needed additional training. Disheartened, Mr. B started to work in a restaurant in a job he felt held no status. He earned enough money to take the additional coursework necessary to apply for a medical license. Mrs. B, on the other hand, did not pursue further professional training here in the United States, and she succeeded in adapting to a low-paying job. During his coursework, Mr. B became increasingly dispirited and discouraged. He could not concentrate on his work or on his schoolwork and failed his exams. He became depressed and constantly irritable with his wife because she appeared happy and content. He began to make more demands on her time and needed her attention constantly. Mrs. B noticed that her husband began to change. He was coming home late at night, and often drunk. She expressed her concern about his condition, and for the first time in their married life, Mr. B slapped her.

Over a period of the next 2 years, Mr. B developed a pattern of drinking every night after work, and his communication with his wife gradually stopped. If at any time she tried to talk to him, he became violent. She began to fear his behavior but did not share this fear with anyone. One night while driving home drunk, he was stopped by a police car and charged with drinking while intoxicated. After his wife paid bail and got him out of jail, he was required to seek treatment and stop his work. Their Asian American family physician suggested a culturally based alcohol treatment program; however, such programs were not available in their town. At this time, Mrs. B found a program that treated women who were victims of domestic violence and started to attend meetings.

Mrs. B's program succeeded in referring her husband to a culturally sensitive Filipino clinician who took an educational approach to Mr. B's alcoholism. He identified the cultural stressors that drove Mr. B to drink, and informed them that alcoholism is a medical condition. He encouraged them to live a healthy lifestyle with diet and exercise and with more involvement in community activities. The clinician additionally recommended the 12-step program offered by Alcoholics Anonymous (AA). Mr. B attended once and refused to return. He could not accept a helplessness approach, although he was able to connect with the spiritual aspect of AA. Mrs. B continued to receive help from the group that assisted victims of domestic violence. In addition, she became involved in Mr. B's treatment, which helped to address family issues and cultural adaptation. Mr. B expressed remorse for his violent behavior toward his wife.

Mr. B's clinician helped him recognize his low self-esteem resulted from his difficulty adjusting to his loss in status in the United States. He displaced his hurt and anger towards his wife. He was also envious that his wife was able to "move on" and adapt to the host culture. Mr. B turned to his spiritual belief system and sought pastoral counseling from his priest. He returned back to work determined to live a healthier, more sober lifestyle.

Summary

1. As in many societies and in many Asian cultures, work is seen as a way to gain status and respect. Mr. B experienced a loss of his social standing when he became underemployed in the United States.
2. Often, the Asian man is expected to be more productive than his spouse. Asian male immigrants may have a difficult time accepting the success of their spouses.
3. Drinking is quite prevalent among Asian immigrants. In some Asian cultures, drinking heavily is culturally accepted. In other cultures, drinking to excess is seen as a negative reflection on the family, so it is often denied or tolerated until it starts to severely impact the proper functioning of a family [7].
4. The intervention for substance abuse should consider the overall well-being of an individual, including a healthy life style, well-balanced diet, and exercise.
5. Asian immigrants may want to incorporate meditation, yoga, or Tai chi into their treatment regimen.
6. Alcoholism is treated as a medical condition, and alternative and holistic treatments such as acupuncture should be prescribed. These treatments may be more acceptable to Asian patients than using only pharmaceutically based treatments.
7. In general, it is critical to follow the patient's lead to explore with the patient their preferred treatment.
8. Many Asian immigrants do not accept self-disclosure in public (e.g., AA). They are more likely to accept individual and family therapy.
9. Domestic violence is not uncommon among Asian Americans and must be handled in a firm but culturally sensitive manner. The clinician may need to educate their patients that domestic violence is not accepted in this culture. It is against the law and is considered a crime.

Case 5: Case of the Stigma of Major Mental Illness

Background and Description of Stressors

Asian American immigrants approach major mental illnesses such as schizophrenia, bipolar disorder, and major depression with psychotic features with denial and secrecy to save the family's reputation. These conditions may bring the entire family dishonor and shame and make it more difficult for the patient as well as for others in the family to find a suitable spouse to marry. Asian

American immigrants tend to tolerate inappropriate behavior and attempt to hide the mentally ill family member to "save face." When efforts to hide the patient fail, the family may first try to medicate the patient with homemade herbal remedies. Next, they might consult a practitioner of traditional medicine or an exorcist before seeking treatment with a psychiatrist. Asian culture may conceptualize hallucinations, delusions, and inappropriate behavior as being caused by the spirit possession from ancestors, evil spirits, and ghosts. Some Asian cultures have a belief in the balance of the five elements (fire, wood, earth, metal, and water) in the Ayurvedic tradition of medicine for a healthy human body. They may also believe in keeping a balance between the good and the evil (Yin and Yang in the Chinese medical tradition) for a healthy mind. Finally, Kapha, Pitta, and Vatta are the three doshas, or dynamic factors, that are considered to be at the core of human functioning in the tradition of Ayurvedic medicine. Kapha corresponds to the solid or the phlegm aspect of the person, Pitta with the fire or fiery aspect of the person, and Vatta with the air or movement aspect of the person. Imbalance of these doshas leads to a disease state. Therefore, all attempts are made to establish a balance of the doshas through traditional and alternative treatments. By the time a hospitalization is indicated, the patient may be very ill, and the family may be in great distress. Clinicians need to approach these patients and their families with cultural sensitivity, the appropriate use of interpreters, and the appropriate use of medications. Finally, educating both the patient and the family about the possible side effects of medications as well as the long-term nature of treatment and the importance of adherence may help to engage the patient in treatment.

Case of Mrs. T

Mrs. T's husband and his aunt brought Mrs. T to the attention of a psychiatrist. They were concerned that she had stopped talking, stopped taking care of her household chores, and performed religious rituals all day long. The patient was mute and unable to engage in the interview. The psychiatrist learned from the husband that the patient's behavior changed 2 years ago, a few months after the family immigrated to the United States from India. She was a soft-spoken woman, who never worked outside the home, and clung to her husband ever since they came to the United States. Her husband noticed that Mrs. T made calls to a priest at odd hours, prayed all the time, and gradually stopped cooking and performing other household chores.

Initially, Mrs. T's husband consulted a traditional practitioner back home who sent some herbal medicines for her. Her husband then involved his aunt who had been in the United States for 10 years. She suggested sending the patient back home to be treated by an exorcist because the patient was talking as if possessed. The patient's husband finally consulted a European American friend who suggested they see a psychiatrist. When her husband learned from the psychiatrist that she needed psychiatric inpatient hospitalization, he panicked. He sought help from her parents but they did not want to be involved for fear that she would spoil the family honor and reputation. They blamed him for her troubles.

After admission to the hospital, Mrs. T was treated with antipsychotic medications, which her husband reluctantly agreed to give her. The patient gradually showed improvement in the hospital. The inpatient psychiatrist educated Mrs. T, her husband, and his aunt about Mrs. T's illness. This involved educating them about the chemical imbalance in the brain causing schizophrenia and the long-term prognosis while also educating them to differentiate between the *behavior* secondary to illness and the *person* as a whole (e.g., her illness did not make her a bad or defective person). The psychiatrist further instilled hope that there were many available treatments and educated them about the importance of adherence with treatment. The husband expressed concerns about the addictive aspects of medications and was concerned that they would bring bodily harm to the patient. After providing appropriate psychoeducation, the psychiatrist recognized the cultural difficulties in treating this patient and asked for the assistance of a South Asian social worker to provide culturally sensitive counseling. The family was pleased to have the opportunity to discuss their concerns in their native language and with someone they felt understood their point of view.

Summary

1. Often, Asian American patients are brought to the clinician's attention after all traditional treatments are exhausted.
2. Family members are often more concerned about family honor, reputation, and stigma than the suffering of an individual.
3. Genetic and psychological causes of schizophrenia may be unacceptable to the family. However, alternative theories, such as the theory of opposite forces causing imbalance of Yin and Yang or imbalance of Kapha, Vatta, and Pitta, may be more acceptable if they carry meaning for the patient.
4. The expression of hallucinations, delusions, and disorganization may be viewed as disruptive to the family's social fabric. Having a relative with mental illness may bring the family shame and dishonor and make it difficult for other family members to find spouses.
5. Medication can be accepted for transient periods, although nonadherence with long-term treatment tends to be very common. Acceptance of alternative treatments in addition to medication may build further trust in the clinician and the medication they prescribe. For illnesses where longer-term medication therapy is warranted, clinicians must continue to build an alliance with the patient and their family, stressing that the patient's well-being will benefit the family.

6. A culturally sensitive clinician must allow the family to express their concerns in addition to educating the patient and family about the importance of treatment.
7. Clinicians must keep in mind that for many Asian immigrants, the family's goal for the treatment of major mental illness (such as schizophrenia) is on restoration of social conformity and function within the family.

Implications for Practice: Specific Subcategories

Asian Americans are the fastest growing racial group in the United States. According to the 2000 census, there are over 10 million Asian Americans, of which 70% are first-generation immigrants [8]. Asian American immigrants face multiple psychosocial stressors, including low socioeconomic status, the loss of an extended family supportive network, the challenge of establishing new social networks, and difficulty with communication in English.

Each Asian immigrant adapts to his or her new culture at a different pace. Educational level, English language proficiency, and employment, in addition to an individual's coping mechanisms, can be important buffers in coping with the stress. Asian immigrants tend to tolerate their feelings of discomfort to a greater degree than many Americans. Families tend to be more accepting of suffering because of their beliefs about paying off karmic debts by accepting an ill family member as a part of their destiny [7]. This serves to make the Asian immigrant more resilient, but can also make them more fatalistic in their attitudes toward life. Inherent in the various stages of acculturation are the possibilities of inter- and intragenerational conflict. Each individual negotiates the two cultures based on one's own cultural beliefs, age at immigration, reasons for the migration, past experiences, internal coping mechanisms, and support from people in the host country. Some variations among gender and various age groups have been identified:

(1) *The Asian woman*. The Asian woman is socialized to be "adaptable." She is socialized to sense quickly what is expected of her under different circumstances and then change her attitude and behave accordingly. She is reared to have her self-esteem based on the approval of others rather than her own achievements. Freedom to think for herself is not encouraged and egalitarian roles are not modeled at home. Women who immigrate as adults with husbands and young children have to renegotiate their identities as career women, wives, and mothers. They struggle with their sense of self as they adjust to a culture very different from that of their childhood.

There is less tolerance for illness in women because her worth is measured in her usefulness to the family. Abandonment of wives whose functioning is not restored as a result of treatment is not uncommon; denial of mental illness by the individuals as well as their families is also very common [5].

(2) *The Asian man.* For the first-generation Asian man, American society not only provides economic opportunity but also challenges the roles at home. Outside factors such as racism, sexism, poverty, and the daily hassles of discrimination add to the experience of stress. Depression, suicide, domestic violence, substance abuse, and even psychotic disorders may manifest. If the wife becomes more successful, the narcissistic injury to the husband may be hard to overcome. Suicide, or murder suicide when a wife leaves or when a job is lost, has been reported in the Indian community newspapers like *India Abroad*. However, in the absence of research studies, these observations are purely anecdotal. Religious beliefs may be a deterrent to suicide; for example, Hindus may assign suffering to previous Karma and destiny, and thus they may be more inclined to accept the suffering and not resort to suicide.

(3) *The Asian Elderly.* These individuals may have been brought to the United States by adult children or they may have immigrated as an older adult. Depending on one's relocation situation in this country, one may feel isolated, exploited, or even held captive. Some Asian elders may feel like a bird that is held captive in a "golden cage" (e.g., possess material luxuries but not the freedom to fly). If they live with their adult children, there may be no places of worship or congregation that they can walk to conveniently and no one to talk to when the adult children are at work. Grandchildren may be ashamed of their grandparents' traditional ways or are unable to speak with them due to language barriers. In addition, independent, assertive, and expressive teenagers may appear offensive to the grandparents. Seeking help is challenging enough, but health insurance may also be a factor. Loss of role, identity, and independence may be too much to bear. As a result, depression may show up for the first time in the older adult's life [4].

(4) *The Asian Youth.* In Asian cultures, there is no clearly identified developmental stage comparable with that of adolescence in the West [9]. In Asia, the emphasis is not on becoming independent from the family of origin but rather on assuming one's role in the family. Many Asian Americans tend to view success or failure based on effort rather than on ability, which further adds to the pressure on the individual. The goals of independent identity formation, deciding on career choice, and deciding on one's life partner (without as much input from the wisdom of nuclear or extended family members) are new experiences for many Asian young adults and their families. Asian youth tend to adapt to the Western culture relatively rapidly. They value the love of their parents but may find themselves in conflict with their parents' wishes regarding careers, life styles, dating, and marriage. They often straddle two cultures and some live dichotomized lives, for example, "all Asian" inside of the home and "all American" outside of the home.

According to the Diagnostic and Statistical Manual-IV, prevalence rates for the major mental illnesses such as schizophrenia and bipolar disorders are the same across all cultures [10]. However, the rates for seeking help, the course of the illness, and the outcomes may be very different. The Asian American as a "model minority," and thus less prone to mental illness is a myth. Asian American individuals and families consistently have lower rates of utilization of psychiatric services [11]. Barriers to seeking help due to stigma and shame continue to challenge Asian Americans. Reluctance to seek help also comes from the lack of recognition of psychiatric problems by both patients and clinicians. Depression can be associated more with themes of shame rather than with guilt, and suicide rates may be higher and related to "failing" the family or not living up to expectations [1, 11, 12].

Treatment: Special Considerations for Psychopharmacological Management

Most Asian American patients enter treatment at later stages of the illness because of all or some of the factors discussed in this chapter. As stated previously, they are likely to be more severely afflicted and become chronically ill by the time they are brought to the attention of a clinician. They may suffer from major psychiatric conditions such as schizophrenia, major depression, PTSD, alcoholism, and anxiety states. Patients may trust the magical curing power of medications, although some may be resistant to the idea of medication management. When medications are accepted as part of a treatment plan, Asian Americans tend to require smaller daily doses of neuroleptics, antidepressants, antimanic agents, and benzodiazepines to achieve steady-state levels, have a more tolerable side effect profile, and optimize treatment [13]. Asian Americans invariably try to self-medicate with herbal treatments, so it is important to take a careful history of any use of vitamins, supplements, and alternative therapies to prevent interactions with Western medicines [14, 15]. It can be noted that some patients may not consider these herbs as medicine and may need psychoeducation. And finally, adherence to medication treatment can be a significant problem because of the patient's belief that short-term treatment leads to a cure. Clinicians must routinely educate the patients about adherence, the course of illness with and without treatment, and explore any undesirable effects that may lead to nonadherence.

Conclusion

The assessment of Asian immigrants must include a cultural formulation, which includes the information that has been highlighted throughout this chapter. Involvement of family is crucial to the successful treatment in most of the patients described in the case scenarios. Family involvement, however, may depend on the level of acculturation of the patient and their family members. Encouraging the patient and family members to express their cultural viewpoints about psychological problems, their past efforts to cope with these problems, and their expectation about treatment is crucial.

Many Asian immigrants tend to place holistic emphasis on the mind–body–spirit connection and believe that individuals react to stress with physical symptoms when the balance between mind, body, and spirit is changed. An effort to conceptualize treatment within the mind–body–spirit continuum may help the patient accept psychological treatment more readily.

Interventions should include consideration of the economic, social, and other essential wellness factors for the patient and the family. Establishing a rapport with the patient may require the clinician to be an advisor, a problem-solver, and possibly an authoritarian figure. The Asian American's individual, family, and community lives are more interwoven if they are more identified with Asian beliefs and values. In these cases, the goal of treatment may not focus on the individual patient's growth but instead focus on an overall harmony in the family and acceptance in the community. Asians are groomed to fit in, and they are expected to do what duty and family honor demands.

These clinical vignettes focus on particular diagnostic, treatment, and therapeutic challenges facing immigrant Asian American individuals and their families. As stated at the beginning of the chapter, these cases represent a sampling of clinical dilemmas and the culturally sensitive approaches to address them. As always, clinicians must begin with cultural hypotheses in treating any patient but must look beyond cultural stereotypes and focus on the particular challenges an individual patient faces. Remembering to truly collaborate with the patient and family while understanding their beliefs about their circumstance and what will help is essential for the successful treatment of these populations.

References

1. Lee E , ed. Working with Asian Americans: A Guide for Clinicians, New York, NY: Guilford Press, 1997.
2. Westermeyer J, ed. Psychiatric Care of the Migrant: A Clinical Guide. Washington, DC: American Psychiatric Press, 1998.
3. Uba L, ed. Asian Americans: Personality Patterns, Identity, and Mental Health. New York, NY: The Guilford Press, 1994.

4. Adler RN and Kamel HK, eds. Doorway Thoughts; Cross Cultural Health Care for Older Adults. Sudbury, MA: Jones and Bartlett Publishers, 2004.
5. Al-Mateen C.S., Christian F.M., Mishra A.S., Cofield M., and Tildon T. Women of Color. In: Kornstein S. and Clayton A., eds. Women's Mental Health. New York, NY: Guilford Press, 2002: 568–583.
6. Westermeyer J, ed. Psychopathology in Psychiatric Care of Immigrants: A Clinical Guide. Washington, DC: American Psychiatric Press, 1989.
7. Ja Y and Yuen F. Substance Abuse Treatment Among Asian Americans. In: Lee E, ed. Working with Asian Americans: A Guide for Clinicians. New York, NY: The Guilford Press, 1997: 295–308.
8. U.S. Bureau of the Census (2001). The Asian American Population (Accessed on March 1 2008, available at http://www.census.gov/population/www/cen2000/briefs.html)
9. Huang LN. Asian American Adolescents. In Lee E ed. Working with Asian Americans; A Guide for Clinicians. New York, NY: The Guilford Press, 1997: 175–195.
10. American Psychiatric Press. Diagnostic and Statistical Manual of Mental Disorders, 4th edn, Text Revision (DSM-IV-TR). Washington DC: American Psychiatric Press, 2000.
11. Sue D and Sue D. Counseling the Culturally Different: Theory and Practice, 2nd edn New York, NY: Wiley Interscience, 1990.
12. Naik US, Menon MS, and Ahmed S. Culture and Psychiatry: An Indian Overview of Issues in Women and Children. In: Okpaku S, ed. Clinical Methods in Transcultural Psychiatry. Washington DC: American Psychiatric Press, 1998: 412–435.
13. Kinzie D and Edeki T. Ethnicity and Psychopharmacology: The Experience of Southeast Asians. In: Okpaku S, ed. Clinical Methods in Transcultural Psychiatry. Washington, DC: American Psychiatric Press, 1998: 171–190.
14. Lininger SW, Austin S, Batz F, and Gaby AR, eds. A–Z Guide to Drug–Herb–Vitamin Interactions: How to Improve Your Health and Avoid Problems when Using Common Medications and Supplements Together. Rocklin, CA, Prima Health, 1999.
15. Pi EH and Gray GE. Ethnopsychopharmacology for Asians. In: Ruiz P ed. Ethnicity and Psychopharmacology. Review of Psychiatry, Volume 19 (4): Washington DC: American Psychiatric Press, 2000: 91–114.

Conclusion

Nhi-Ha Trinh and Yanni Rho

Acculturation, as we have seen, is a multidimensional process, impacting Asian American individuals, their families, and their communities. Researchers continue to develop methods to better study acculturation in Asian Americans, including developing refined ways of measurement, refining outcomes, and investigating implications for Asian American health. In addition, newer concepts such as enculturation and the parent–child acculturation gap, as well as new interventions, enable researchers to develop a more nuanced view of how acculturation affects Asian American immigrants and their families.

This research has many implications for clinical practice. By incorporating a cultural formulation model, epidemiologic studies, and increased understanding of the process of acculturation on families, we will be more reflective in our approach to individual patients. Understanding the particular sociohistorical context of Asian American groups as well as the personal and individual contexts of their lives is an invaluable part of the evaluation and treatment of our patients. This will be true whether we are dealing with a college student struggling with anxiety over academic achievement, an Asian American family coping with a grandparent with dementia, or a Southeast Asian refugee coping with trauma and posttraumatic stress disorder. Furthermore, theory and research is only part of the story; its translation into our thoughtful clinical work and continued enthusiasm for learning from patients is fundamental. For example, the cases provided by our authors illustrate the complexities that arise, as we try to understand the individual with their cultural and social context.

As the Asian American population in the United States acculturates into the proverbial "melting pot," several issues will become more important to address in the coming decades. These include understanding resiliency in acculturation, tackling enculturation as well as acculturation issues in multiple-generation Asian Americans, understanding the impact of interethnic/interracial marriage, bi- and multiracial/ethnic heritage, and the impact of Asian adoption on Asian

N.-H. Trinh (✉)
Massachusetts General Hospital, Depression Clinical Research Program, Boston MA, USA
e-mail: ntrinh@partners.org

American cultural identity. What it means to be Asian American will inevitably change.

In sum, this volume both proposes and challenges cultural hypotheses. It is not meant to be a prescriptive, encyclopedic "how-to" guide. We hope to challenge readers to reflect not only on the dynamic process of acculturation for Asian Americans but also on how acculturation theories may be applicable to other ethnic groups. Learning to take better care of Asian American patients will ultimately translate into taking better care of all our patients. Regardless of specific background, our struggle to make sense of our cultural and ethnic identity is ultimately universal.

Index

A

Acculturation
    assessment of, 5–8
    case studies, 180–195
    construct definitions of, 26–28
    defined, 4–5
    future research recommendations, 65–74
    identifying phase of, 72
    rates for individual Asian American family members, 103
    state of disequilibrium, 105
    status and its affects, 8–18
Acculturation, Habits, and Interests Multicultural Scale for Adolescents (AHIMSA), 8
The Acculturation Scale, 7
Acculturation stressors
    alcoholism/domestic violence/ intragenerational stress (case study), 188–190
    conflict secondary to intra- and intergenerational acculturation (case study), 180–183
    generalized anxiety and panic attacks (case study), 183–185
    implication for clinical practices, 192–194
    psychopharmacological management, 194–195
    somatization of attitudes toward mental health treatment based on degree of acculturation (case study), 185–187
    stigma of major mental illness (case study), 190–192
Acculturative Family Distancing (AFD), 28–29
Acculturative stress, 11–13, 29
Adaptation
    exigency stage, 83–84
    marginality acceptance, phase of, 84
    resolution stage, 84
    social marginality, phase of, 84
    of Southeast Asian population in United States, 128–132
Adolescents
    Asian American, *see* Asian American adolescents/children
    immigrants, identity formation issues, 104
Alcohol consumption
    acculturation status and, 11
    alcoholisms (case study), 188–190
Anxiety
    in Asian American children/adolescents, 152–153
    case study, 183–185
    risk in Asian American elderly population, 169–170
Asian American adolescents/children
    anxiety in, 152–153
    clinical considerations, 145–146, 146–148
    general thoughts, 159–161
    delinquency and gang-related activity of, 155–156
    depression in, 151–152
    generational/cultural gap, 148
    ego identity in, 147–148
    evaluation and treatment of, 159
    identity formation in adolescent immigrants, 104, 147–148
    importance of acculturation assessment, 148–149
    parental psychopathology impact, 149–150
    psychopathology in, 151–158
    risk factors and resiliency, 158–159
    somatized distress, in, 151
    substance abuse in, 154–155
    working with, 161–162

Asian American elderly
  anxiety risk in, 169–170
  caregiving for, 174–175
  death rate, 168
  dementia in, 172–173
  future directions and clinical implications for, 175–176
  growth rate, 168
  risk of depression and anxiety in, 169–170
  suicide risk in, 170–172
Asian American families, 25–26
  acculturation, 101–105
    cultural conflict, 112
    development, 103–104
    family dynamics, 102–103
    family ecologies, 104–105
    family structure, 103
  acculturation and enculturation for, 26–32
    constructs of, 26–28
    theories and research on consequences of, 28–32
  acculturation assessment, 106–117
    in couple subsystem, 112–117
    in parent–child subsystem, 106–112
  child–parent cultural values gap and intergenerational conflicts, 32–41
  impact of American culture, 102
  mental health, 81–94
    acculturation stress, 83–84
    epidemiology of, 87–93
    key factors affecting, 85–87
    services, usage of, 93
  as "model minority", 84
  parent–child communication, 102–103
  within-group diversity, 82–83
Asian American Multidimensional Acculturation Scale (AAMAS), 7
Asian Pacific American LGBTI youth, identity complexity, 157–158
Asian values gap, child–parent, intergenerational conflicts and, 32–41
Asian Values Scale (AVS), 6
Asian Values Scale – Revised (AVS-R), 34
Assimilation, acculturation outcome, 4
"Attachment anxiety," 12

B
Behavioral acculturation, *versus* values acculturation, 71–72
Behavioral acculturation scales, 5–6
  values, combined with, 7

Biculturalism, 8, 30, 73, 109, 180
Boat people, 127

C
Cambodians, in United States, 125, 127–128
Canadian National Population Health survey, 9
Career decisions, acculturation status and, 15–16
Caregiving, for Asian American elderly, 174–175
Central Intelligence Agency (CIA) during Vietnam War, 126, 128
Children
  Asian American, *see* Asian American adolescents/children
  See also Parent–child conflicts; Parent–child cultural values gap
Chinese American immigrants
  SITIF's effectiveness with, 50–62
    discussion, 59–62
    method, 52–55
    results, 56–59
Chinese American Psychiatric Epidemiological Study (CAPES), 91
Chinese-Vietnamese refugee, 127
Church World Service, 129
Cognitive flexibility, 28–29
  and parent–child conflicts, 30
    cultural values gap, relationship with, 32–41
Cognitive Flexibility Scale (CFS), 34–35
Communication competence, 40
Conflicts
  cultural, in Asian American families, 112
  family practices leading to, 106–107
  family values and, 106–107
  parent–child, *see* Parent–child conflicts
Constructs of acculturation/enculturation, 26
Coronary heart disease, acculturation status and, 9
Counseling process, acculturation status and attitude towards, 16–18
Couple dynamics, Asian American families, 114–115
Couple subsystem, acculturation assessment, 112–117
  change in gender attitudes and roles, 112–113
  changes in couple dynamics and risk for domestic abuse, 114–115

developmental considerations, 115–116
ethnic minority status and transnational family ecologies in, 116–117
status inconsistency, 113–114
    questions to assess, 114
Cultural conflicts, in Asian American families, 112
"Cultural maintenance", 26–27
Cultural values gap, parent–child intergenerational conflicts and, 32–41
    instruments, 33–35
    limitations and implications, 40–41
    method, 33
    procedure, 35–36
    results, 36–40
"Culture conflict model", 29

D
Delinquency, Asian American adolescents/children, 155–156
Dementia, in Asian American elderly, 172–173
    epidemiology, 172–173
    family perception, 173
Demographic shifts, in Asian American elderly population, 168
Depression
    acculturation status and, 12–13
    in Asian American children/adolescents, 151–152
    generational/cultural gap, 148
    impact on Asian American parents, 150
    risk in Asian American elderly population, 169–170
    suicide, risk factor, 93
Developmental age, identifying study populations by individual characteristics, 69–70
Diagnostic and Statistical Manual, Fourth Edition (DSM-IV), 169–170
Directive counseling approach, 17
Discrimination, 87
Dispersion, systematic, Southeast Asian refugees, 131–132
"Dissonant acculturation", 29
Domestic violence, 86–87
    in Asian American families, 114–115
    case study, 187–190
DSM-IV, *see* Diagnostic and Statistical Manual, Fourth Edition (DSM-IV)

E
Eating disorders, acculturation status and, 9–10
Economic status, Southeast Asian refugees, 131
Ego identity, in Asian American adolescents, 147–148
Elderly, Asian American, *see* Asian American elderly
Emotional expression, 107–109
Enculturation
    for Asian American families, 26–32
    construct definitions of, 26–28
Epidemiological Catchment Area (ECA) study, 90–91
Ethnic identity, 147
    identification of study population by group, 67–68
Ethnic minority status, Asian American families, 105
    in couple acculturation, 116–117
European Americans *versus* Korean Americans, 158–159
European American Values Scale for Asian Americans (EAVS-AA), 6–7
European American Values Scale for Asian Americans – Revised, 41
Exigency stage, adaptation, 83–84
Externalized behaviors, of Asian American adolescents/children, 155–156

F
Family dynamics, Asian American families acculturation, 102–103
Family ecology, Asian American families acculturation, 104–105
    effects of transnational, 105
    ethnic minority status, 105
Family role
    acculturation status and adjustment, 13
    conflicts
        intergenerational, *see* Intergenerational conflicts
        practices leading to, 106–107
        values and, 106–107
    identification of study population by group, 68–69
    perceptions of dementia, in Asian American elderly, 173
Family structure, Asian American families acculturation, 103
Filial therapy, 49

G

Gang-related activity, of Asian American children/adolescents, 155–156
Gender role
  Asian American families
    gender attitudes in, 112–113
    gender issues in, 157–158
  in career decision-making self-efficacy, 16
  identifying study populations by individual characteristics, 70
  parent–child conflicts and, 31
Generational/cultural gap, in Asian Americans, 148–149
Glass ceiling effect, 30

H

Hwa-Byung (HB), 82

I

Identifying study populations
  by groups, 67–69
  by individual characteristics, 69–70
Identity, ethnic, identification of study population by group, 67–68
Identity, of Asian American population
  ego identity in adolescents, 147–148
  formation in adolescent immigrants, 104, 147–148
Identity, sexual, 157–158
Identity crisis, 86
Identity development, new, 84
Immigrants
  Chinese American, *see* Chinese American immigrants
  identification of study population by group, 68
  identity formation in Asian American adolescents, 104, 147–148
  See also Strengthening Intergenerational/Intercultural Ties in Immigrant Families (SITIF)
Instrumentation, 71
Integration, acculturation outcome, 4
Interethnic dating, Asian Americans, 156–158
Intergenerational Conflict Inventory (ICI), 35
Intergenerational conflicts, 85–86
  parent–child cultural values gap and, 32–41
  See also Strengthening Intergenerational/Intercultural Ties in Immigrant Families (SITIF)

Intraethnic differences, 68
Intragenerational stress, case study, 188–190
IUS (Involvement in the American culture) score, 7
IVN (Involvement in the Vietnamese culture) score, 7

K

Korean Americans *versus* European Americans, 158–159, 174

L

Laotians, in United States, 125, 128
Lesbian, gay, bisexual, transgender, and intersexual (LGBTI), 157–158
LGBTI, *see* Lesbian, gay, bisexual, transgender, and intersexual (LGBTI)
Lutheran Immigration and Refugee Service, 129

M

Marginality acceptance, adaptation phase, 84
Marginalization, acculturation outcome, 5
"Marginalized" person, 73
Marin Acculturation Scale, 6
Measurement procedure issues, acculturation, 71–73
Mental health
  acculturation status and, 11–13
  Asian American families, 81–94
    acculturation stress, 83–84
    epidemiology of, 87–93
    issues in elderly population, 169–173
    key factors affecting, 85–87
    mental health services, usage of, 93
  case studies, 186–187, 190–192
  issues in Southeast Asian refugees, 134–137
Migration history, Southeast Asian population, 125–128
Minority status, ethnic, 105
"Model minority", Asian American families as, 84
Multicultural Acculturation Scale (MAS), 8
Multiracial heritage, identifying study populations by individual characteristics, 70

Index

N
National Comorbidity Study (NCS), 90–91
National Latino and Asian American Study, 91
National Youth Tobacco Survey (NYTS), 154
New identity, development, 84
Nondirective counseling approach, 17
NYTS, *see* National Youth Tobacco Survey (NYTS)

O
Obesity, acculturation status and, 9–10
Objective mastery of SITIF curriculum, 54–55, 56–57, 60–61
Orthogonal Cultural Identification Scale, 8
Orthogonal scales, 5, 72–73

P
Pan-ethnic acculturation scales, 7–8
Panic attacks, case study, 183–185
Parental overprotection, 31–32
Parental psychopathology, Asian American adolescents, 149–150
Parent–child communication, Asian American families, 102–103
　conflicts over, 107–109
Parent–child conflicts, 28–32
　cognitive flexibility and, 30
　　cultural values gap, relationship with, 32–41
　communication related, Asian American families, 107–109
　cultural values gap and intergenerational conflicts, 32–41
　gender role in, 31
　over family practices and values, 106–107
　questions to assess, 107
　See also Conflicts
Parent–child cultural values gap
　intergenerational conflicts and, 32–41
　　instruments, 33–35
　　limitations and implications, 40–41
　　method, 33
　　procedure, 35–36
　　results, 36–40
Parent–child relationships change, in SE Asian refugees, 133–134
Parent–child subsystem, acculturation assessment, 106–112
　conflicts, 106–109
　　over communication and emotional expression, 107–109
　　over family practices and values, 106–107
　differential experiences of acculturation, 109–110
　role reversals in, 110–111
　significance of exosystems and mesosystems, 112
Parent's role
　engagement with SITIF, 54, 56, 59–60
　in school performance, 14
Personality, identifying study populations by individual characteristics, 69
Physical health, acculturation status and, 9–11
Posttraumatic stress disorder (PTSD), in Southeast Asian refugees, 136–137
Prejudice, 87
Pre-migration traumatic experiences (PTE), 84
Psychological acculturation, 26
Psychological distress, acculturation status and, 11–12
Psychopathology, Asian American adolescents, 151–158
　parental, impacts, 149–150
　somatized distress, 151
Psychopharmacological management, acculturation stressors, 195
Psychotherapy process, acculturation status and attitude towards, 16–18
PTSD, *see* Posttraumatic stress disorder (PTSD), in Southeast Asian refugees

R
Refugee Services of US Catholic Conferences, 129
Religious organization, assistance to Southeast Asian refugees, 129
Research recommendations, future
　design considerations, 73–74
　identifying study populations, 67–70
　measurement procedure issues, 71–73
Resettlement, of Southeast Asian population in United States, 128–132
Resolution stage, adaptation, 84
Role reversals, in parent–child subsystem, 110–111

S
Scales, acculturation measure
　behavioral, 5–6
　combined (behavioral and values), 7

Scales, acculturation measure (*cont.*)
  orthogonal, 5, 72–73
  Pan-ethnic, 7–8
  values, 6–7
School performance
  acculturation status and, 14–15
  parent's role in, 14
Scores, *see* Scales, acculturation measure
Separation, acculturation outcome, 4
Sexual identity, 157–158
Sexuality, Asian Americans, 157–158
SITIF, *see* Strengthening Intergenerational/
    Intercultural Ties in Immigrant
    Families (SITIF)
Smoking behaviors, acculturation status
    and, 10–11
Social marginality, adaptation phase, 84
Social network, change in Southeast Asian
    refugees, 132–134
Somatized distress, in Asian American
    adolescents/children, 151
Southeast Asian families, change in, 132–134
Southeast Asian refugees
  from Cambodia, 127–128
  changes in social network and, 132–134
    parent–child relationships, 133–134
    traditional multigenerational pattern
      of kinship, 132
  Chinese-Vietnamese refugee, 127
  clinical practice with, 137–138
  economic status, 131
  impact of American culture, 130
  from Laos, 128
  mental health issues, 134–137
    posttraumatic stress disorder (PTSD),
      136–137
    traumatic events, 134–135
  premigration and migration history,
    125–128
  reception by US communities, 131
  religious organization and, 129
  resettlement and adaptation in United
    States, 128–132
  serach for employment, 130–131
  systematic dispersion, 131–132
  in United States, 124–125
  from Vietnam, 127
Southeast Asian veterans, of Vietnam
    War, 113
Status inconsistency, Asian American
    families, 114–115

Stephenson Multigroup Acculturation
    Scale, 7
Strengthening Intergenerational/
    Intercultural Ties in Immigrant
    Families (SITIF), 46–47
  Chinese American immigrants,
    effectiveness in, 50–62
    discussion, 59–62
    method, 52–55
    results, 56–59
  description of, 48–50
  significance of, 47–48
Stress, acculturative, 11–13, 29
  Asian American mental health, 83–84
Study populations, identification
  by groups, 67–69
  by individual characteristics, 69–70
Subjective evaluation of SITIF's
    effectiveness, 55, 57–59, 61
Substance abuse, Asian American children/
    adolescents, 154–155
Suicide
  acculturation status and, 12–13
  depression, risk factor for, 93
  risk in Asian American elderly
    population, 170–172
  risk in Asian American youths, 153–154
Suinn–Lew Asian Self-Identity Acculturation
    Scale (SL-ASIA), 5–6
"Suppressed anger syndrome", 82

V

Values acculturation, behavioral
    acculturation *versus,* 71–72
Values acculturation scales, 6–7
  behavior, combined with, 7
Vietnamese, in United States, 124–125, 127
Vietnam War, 125, 126
  Southeast Asian refugees and, 131, 135
  Southeast Asian veterans of, 113
VOLAG, *see* Voluntary Resettlement
    Agencies (VOLAG)
Voluntary Resettlement Agencies
    (VOLAG), 129

W

World Relief Refugee Services of the
    National Association of World
    Evangelicals, 129

Printed in the United States of America